Manual Medicine
Diagnostics

Manual Medicine
Diagnostics

Jiří Dvořák and Václav Dvořák

With the Collaboration of Tomáš Drobný
Translated and edited by
Wolfgang G. Gilliar and Philip E. Greenman
Forewords by Mark Mumenthaler and Barry D. Wyke
175 Mostly Colored Figures, 6 Tables

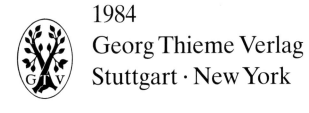

1984
Georg Thieme Verlag   Thieme-Stratton Inc.
Stuttgart · New York   New York

Jiří Dvořák MD
Dept. of Neurology, University Hospital
Inselspital
CH-3010 Berne, Switzerland

Václav Dvořák MD
General Practitioner
CH-7402 Bonaduz, Switzerland

Tomáš Drobný MD
Dept. of Orthopedics of the Surgical Clinic
Kantonsspital Bruderholz
CH-4101 Bruderholz, Switzerland

Translators:
Wolfgang G. Gilliar, B.S.
Philip E. Greenman, D.O.
Michigan State University
College of Osteopathic Medicine
Office of the Dean
East Fee Hall
East Lansing, MI 48823, USA

This book is an authorized translation from the German edition published and copyrighted 1983 by Georg Thieme Verlag, Stuttgart, West Germany.
Title of the German edition:
Manuelle Medizin – Diagnostik

Deutsche Bibliothek Cataloguing in Publication Data

Dvořák, Jiří:
Manual medicine : diagnostics / Jiří Dvořák and Václav Dvořák. With the collab. of Tomáš Drobný. Transl. by Wolfgang G. Gilliar and Philip E. Greenman. Forewords by Mark Mumenthaler and Barry D. Wyke. – Stuttgart ; New York : Thieme ; New York : Thieme-Stratton, 1984.
  Deutsche Ausg. u.d.T.: Dvořák, Jiří: Manuelle Medizin

NE: Dvořák, Václav:

Important Note: Medicine is an ever-changing science. Research and clinical experience are continually broadening our knowledge, in particular our knowledge of proper treatment and drug therapy. Insofar as this book mentions any dosage or application, readers may rest assured that the authors, editors and publishers have made every effort to ensure that such references are strictly in accordance with the state of knowledge at the time of production of the book. Nevertheless, every user is requested to carefully examine the manufacturer's leaflets accompanying each drug to check on his own responsibility whether the dosage schedules recommended therein or the contraindications stated by the manufacturers differ from the statements made in the present book. Such examination is particularly important with drugs which are either rarely used or have been newly released on the market.

© 1984 Georg Thieme Verlag, Rüdigerstrasse 14, D-7000 Stuttgart 30, West Germany
Printed in West Germany
Typesetting (System 5, Linotron 202) by Druckhaus Dörr, D-7140 Ludwigsburg
Printed by K. Grammlich, Pliezhausen

ISBN 3-13-624601-2 (Georg Thieme Verlag, Stuttgart)
ISBN 0-86577-124-3 (Thieme Stratton Inc., New York)
LOC 84-051390

Foreword

The undersigned has neither received a formal education in manual therapy, nor does he practice such (this sentence is not a pleonasm!). Furthermore, he is neither disappointed by his own field or frustrated because of other reasons. When he recommended that this book should appear at all, this was not due to personal or complex-psychological motives, nor an innate trust in this form of medicine itself.

The reasons are, on the contrary, quite rational. As a recent poll by the Swiss Medical Society for Manual Medicine indicated, approximately 300,000 manipulations are performed by physicians in Switzerland every year. About 100 chiropractors manipulate nearly 800,000 times per year. This amounts to a total of some 1.1 million manipulations in Switzerland every year. We neurologists especially, however, tend to see the undesirable side effects and complications of manual medicine. Is this therefore not enough reason in itself to recommend a thorough explanation of one of the techniques and its fundamentals? Further, the author of this foreword has been privileged to have had numerous personal contacts with non-medical chiropractors and physicians practicing manual medicine who have demonstrated responsible and ethically irreproachable attitude, in depth training and convincing therapeutic success. This alone would be a good reason for a representative of formal, organized medicine to support a publication which advocates manual therapy.

On the other hand, one experiences in diverse discussions, as always in this field, that one school of thought is set against another, when irrational and unverifiable elements with confusing terminology come into play; actually, therapeutic acts begin to assume the form of pure magic! The beneficial effects of this therapy became simply a "last resort", albeit obligatory, alternative for treatment due to the ubiquitous prejudicial consensus of opinion concerning this form of medicine. Patient demands, however, or official control forced many therapists into a sterile confinement and restricted them in every case which presented itself into using this single approach in a one-sided intractability. A further reason in this respect for publishing one of these methods of treatment was the need for a clear and unambiguous statement of principles, claims and limitations.

This leads to the fourth and probably the most important reason for this publication: even though manual therapy has developed empirically, as indeed today's medicine has originally developed, it might nevertheless fulfill some of the patients' expectations by a direct, "close-hand" approach which corresponds to their wishes for a "magical" panacea. With its own intrinsic procedures, manual therapy can further be viewed as a challenge to the technical and impersonal aspects of modern medicine. All this, however, is not a reason to not subject manual medicine to scientific methodology. In this context, the term "scientific" implies:

– building on existing foundations, identifying the tangible phenomena, and
– making these comprehensible and learnable.

Many representatives of this type of treatment and other "alternatives" to formal medicine have largely evaded any meaningful discussion of their particular field of activity, when brought to task. Usually, they shelter behind a mass of esoteric terminology and avoid a rational promulgation of their fundamentals, preventing them from being studied.

The physicians Jiří Dvořák, who has a comprehensive knowledge of general medicine as well as a training in neurology, Václav Dvořák, trained in internal medicine, and Tomáš Drobný, with a surgical and orthopedic specialist training behind him, have all worked as students under the auspices of the internal specialist Max Sutter as well as pursuing their own interest in manual medicine. They were thus presented with the opportunity not only to demonstrate their reproducible successes in therapeutics, but also had the courage to establish the scientific basis of the principles pertaining thereto, and lay these open to discussion. They have done this knowing that the last word in this matter has not yet been reached. They would like their interpretation of the mechanisms of manual medicine to be scrutinized, challenged and perhaps corrected. To this end it is essential that the subject be candidly laid bare. Only in this respect is the chance presented for the material to become useful and valid in the long term. To this effect, this book is scientific.

Bern   MARK MUMENTHALER

Foreword

Articular neurology is the branch of neurology that is concerned with the morphology, physiology, pathology, and clinical features of the innervation of the joints of the body (including those in the vertebral column), but until about 15 years ago this discipline did not exist as an organized body of knowledge, since it had never been studied systematically in the laboratory or the clinic. Happily, articular neurology has now been developed to the point where it forms one of the basic sciences of orthopedic medicine and surgery, as well as of clinical neurology.

The observations reported in this monograph represent an important clinical application of some of what is now known of articular reflexology in a diagnostic context, and as such should prove to be of considerable significance to practitioners of manual medicine and physical therapy, as well as of orthopedics, rheumatology, and neurology. For too long, manual medicine has existed as an empirical art rather than as a clinical science, but this monograph – based as it is on some of the scientific data currently available in the field of articular neurology – should go some way toward remedying this state of affairs. It therefore gives me considerable pleasure to contribute this foreword to a work that I hope will serve as a stimulus to clinicians in a variety of disciplines, as well as to practitioners of manual medicine.

London

Prof. Dr. B. D. WYKE, M.D., B.S.
Director of the Neurological Unit,
Royal College of Surgeons of England

Preface

The ever-increasing interest in manual medicine has encouraged us to present this review of the methods and techniques currently used in this field, be they of general or specific diagnostic value. This book was written with both the general practitioner and the physician specializing in manual medicine in mind. In addition to presenting the biomechanics and the functional examination of the vertebral column, we have tried to correlate alterations in the soft tissues that cause pain (nonradicular spondylogenic syndromes) – which are so far only known emperically – with findings in basic research of the neurophysiological processes. In this sense, it seems only natural to begin by correlating the practical experiences gained through patient examination with the results of neurophysiological research concerning the phenomenon of pain. This correlation of clinical observations with experimental findings will perhaps stimulate further research of pain syndromes the causes of which are often unknown and that may pose a central problem to the physician using manual techniques.

We have deliberately excluded the radiology of the vertebral column and the orthopedic, rheumatological, and neurophysiological examinations, since they appear in the classic literature. It goes without saying that a differential diagnosis in manual medicine should be made in accordance with the standards of modern-day practice of the medical profession.

The physician is often confronted with patients who present with pain of unknown origin, which is known as "noninflammatory soft tissue rheumatism." Chapters 7 and 10 attempt to catalogue these painful syndromes and correlate them with the skeleton. They are based on observations made by Dr. M. Sutter, who has examined a large number of patients. His main contribution was to understand that painful syndromes arising from the spine and the extremities could be identified and correlated with the anatomy. This in turn determines the therapeutic approach – manual therapy being one of the choices. We are deeply indebted to Dr. Sutter for his extensive palpatory studies done over many years, as well as for his knowledge in this field. We

had the opportunity of working closely with him between 1976 and 1979. Dr. Sutter's teaching presented us with the opportunity of working in the area of the "spondylogenic reflex syndromes" and subsequently to develop this review.

We also want to thank Prof. K. Ludwig and his coworkers Dr. Bauer and Dr. Schwitzgebel from the Anatomy Institute of the University in Basle for helpful suggestions and corrections. We would also thank Prof. M. Mumenthaler of the Neurological Department of the University Hospital in Berne for his help in preparing this book. We thank Prof. B. D. Wyke and his coworkers from the Neurological Unit of the Royal College of Surgeons of England, whose neurophysiological findings became the basis for the understanding of the spondylogenic reflex syndrome. Dr. Wyke's critical, yet encouraging, instructions inspired us to continue research in this field. With the kind permission of Prof. A. White, Harvard Medical School, and Prof. M. Panjabi, Yale University, we were able to use a number of illustrations depicted in their book, Clinical Biomechanics of the Spine, to clarify concepts in our chapters on the biomechanics of the vertebral column.

We would further like to mention our appreciation to Prof. P. E. Greenman, Michigan State University, College of Osteopathic Medicine, for his cooperation, invaluable suggestions, and his help in getting this book published and translated into English language.

Translating a work such as this is no easy task, especially when the terminology is subject to variation in both languages. Wolfgang Gilliar with his diligence and great interest in the subject matter has mastered this task. We thank him for the precision of his translation of the text.

Last, yet not least, we would like to thank Georg Thieme Verlag and Thieme-Stratton Inc. Special thanks are extended to Dr. D. Bremkamp and Mr. A. Menge for their cooperation as well as to everyone, even though not mentioned individually, who made this project feasible.

Berne and Bonaduz,
September 1984

Jiří Dvořák
Václav Dvořák

Contents

1. Biomechanics and Functional Examination of the Vertebral Column

An understanding of the biomechanics of the spinal column is indispensable, not only for examination procedures, but also for the evaluation of roentgenograms and therapy. In this chapter therefore we place emphasis on the biomechanics based on the fundamental work by WHITE and PANJABI, 1978a and b. Described are only those methods of examination that, in addition to rheumatological, orthopedic, and neurological procedures, have proved to be useful.

1.1. Occipital-Atlanto-Axial Complex

1.1.1. Atlanto-Occipital Joint

The articulation between the skull and the atlas is formed by two paired structures, each pair consisting of the occipital condyle and the superior facets of the atlas. The articulating surfaces are oval, sometimes showing a beanlike configuration. The upper surface of the condyles is convex, and the surface of the superior facets of the atlas is concave. The sagittal axial angle of the joints is 50° to 60° for the adult (INGELMARK, 1947; BERNHARD, 1976) (Fig. 1).

The frontal axial angle of the joints (Fig. 2) results from lines drawn parallel to the articulating surfaces of the condyles. On the average, it is 124.2°

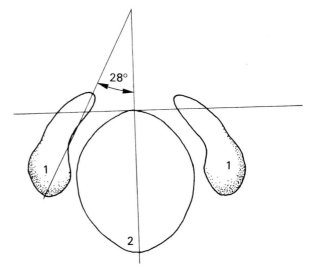

Fig. 1. Sagittal angle of the joint axes for the occipital condyles (after *Ingelmark*, 1947). 1: occipital condyles; 2: foramen magnum.

(STOFF, 1976). This axial angle increases in the event of condylar hypoplasia and basilar impression.

VON LANZ and WACHSMUTH (1979) describe the joint between the skull and the atlas as a modified spherical articulation, with mobility about two axes according to the anatomical arrangement. The left and right joints acting in conjunction allow move-

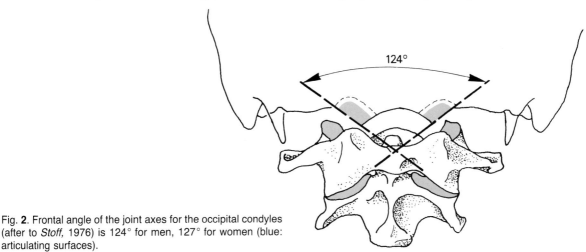

Fig. 2. Frontal angle of the joint axes for the occipital condyles (after to *Stoff*, 1976) is 124° for men, 127° for women (blue: articulating surfaces).

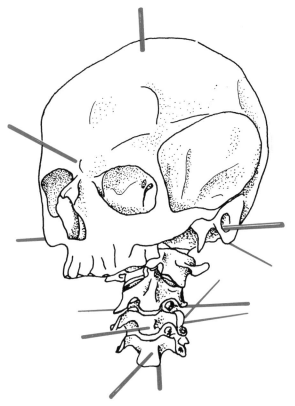

Fig. 3. Axes of motion of the occipital-atlanto-axial and cervical joints (after *Knese*, 1947/50).

ment about the larger transverse axis and the smaller sagittal axis.

Flexion and extension movements take place about the transverse axis, whereas lateral bending is about the sagittal axis (Fig. 3).

Function of the Atlanto-Occipital Joint

Flexion and extension (about the transverse axis), which ranges between 16° and 20°, is limited by the

Table 1   Restriction of the Range of Motion of the Occipital-Atlanto-Axial Joints about the Transverse Axis

Flexion	Extension
Nuchal ligament	Bony limitation
Posterior longitudinal ligament	Anterior muscles of the back
Longitudinal fasciculus of the cruciform ligament	Aponeurosis of the biceps brachii muscle
Tectorial membrane	Alar ligaments
Posterior muscles of the back	Anterior longitudinal ligament

bony structures and the surrounding functional soft tissue (Table 1).

Lateralbending about the sagittal axis measures 4° to either side. When the head is in a slightly flexed position, lateral bending reaches a maximum; when extended, such bending is prohibited by the alar ligaments.

Different data exist in the literature in regard to the rotation of the atlanto-occipital joint: FIELDING (1957, 1978), WHITE and PANJABI (1978a and b), and PENNING (1968) found no rotation, whereas DEPREUX and MESTDAGH (1974) contend that a rotation of 5° exists, which can increase substantially after atlanto-axial fusion. CAVIEZEL (1976) clinically examines the "passive terminal rotation" of the atlas in the test of resiliency.

1.1.2. Atlantoaxial Joint

The atlantoaxial joint is very important for manual medicine. Motion takes place in four articular spaces, one of which is designated the bursa atlantodentalis; this is the space between the transverse ligament of the atlas and the dens of the axis.

The middle atlantoaxial joint is located between the dens of the axis and the posterior surface of the anterior arch of the atlas. The two articular spaces of the lateral atlantoaxial joint are of primary importance. The joint surfaces are usually round, sometimes triangular and covered with cartilage of 1.4 to 3.2 mm thickness. The articular surfaces of the axis are convex, and those of the atlas are relatively flat, causing an anterior and posterior gap of 2 to 5 mm (KNESE, 1947/50) (Fig. 4). The joint capsule is wide and flabby, and from the medial wall a cuneiform synovial fold reaches into the articular space (meniscoid).

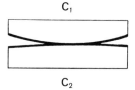

Fig. 4. Schematic representation of the articulating surfaces of atlas and axis.

Function of the Atlantoaxial Joints

Flexion/extension: The bony structures of the articular surfaces along with the securing ligamentous apparatus allow only minimal movement about the transverse axis of not more than 10 to 15°, (Fig. 3). In the lateral x-ray, the effectiveness of the ligaments can be determined by the distance between the back of the anterior arch of the atlas and the dens of the axis. As this distance increases, so does insufficiency.

Lateral flexion: Lateral bending between C_1 and C_2 is only possible with simultaneous rotation about the axis.

This is described as forced rotation and is mainly the result of the physiological function of the alar ligaments. LEWIT (1970) and JIROUT (1973) report dislocation of the atlas in the direction of the bending when lateralbending is forced.

Rotation: The head and atlas rotate simultaneously on the axis about the dens. The rotational axis passing through the dens of the axis is determined by the transverse ligament of the atlas (Fig. **3**). The range of motion to each side is normally 40° to 50°, which is about half of the total cervical spine rotation. Kinematographic studies by FIELDING (1957, 1978) clearly demonstrate that starting from the neutral position rotation takes place in the atlantoaxial joints first. Once their motion is completed, the lower cervical spine segments begin to rotate. The limitation of the rotation is primarily effected by the alar ligaments (Figs. **6, 7**).

1.1.3. Ligaments of the Occipital-Atlanto-Axial Complex

In this context, only those ligaments are described that appear important for the function of the atlanto-occipital and atlanto-axial joints, such as the alar ligaments and the cruciform ligament of the atlas.

Alar Ligaments

LUDWIG (1952) describes the alar ligament as an irregular, quadrilateral pyramid-like trunk. The rectangular base lies against the superior two-thirds of the lateral surface of the dens. The superior, posterior and anterior surfaces connect the dens with the occipital condyle, and the inferior and lateral surfaces connect the dens with the lateral mass of the atlas (Fig. **5**).

Function of the Alar Ligaments

During extension of the head, the alar ligament is stretched, whereas during flexion it is relaxed.

During rotation of the atlantoaxial joint, the ligament of the opposite side is stretched and "rolled up" around the dens of the axis; the ligament on the same side relaxes. Thus, during rotation to the right, the left alar ligament is "rolled up", and the right ligament relaxes (Fig. **6**).

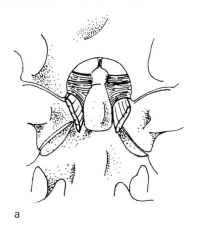

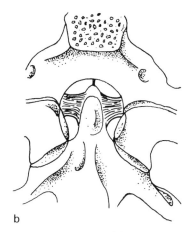

a

b

Fig. **5**. Alar ligaments: **(a)** posterior view, **(b)** anterior view (after *Ludwig*, 1952).

During bending to one side, the alar ligament of that same side relaxes, and the stretched ligament of the opposite side causes a forced rotation of the axis in the direction of the bending due to the attachment to the dens of the axis (the spinous process of the axis moves contralaterally; Fig. **7**). Thus, the strong alar ligaments are able to limit the rotation of the atlantoaxial joints.

Cruciform Ligament of the Atlas

The cruciform ligament consists of the horizontal transverse ligament of the atlas and the vertical longitudinal fasciculi. The transverse ligament of the atlas arises from the medial surfaces of the lateral masses of the atlas, portions of the fibers being attached to the tip of the dens. The ligament consists primarily of collagen fibers that can be irreversibly stretched under strong tension (KENNEDY et al., 1976). The central portion of the ligament is 10 mm high, 2 mm thick, and covered by a thin layer of cartilage. The longitudinal fasciculi

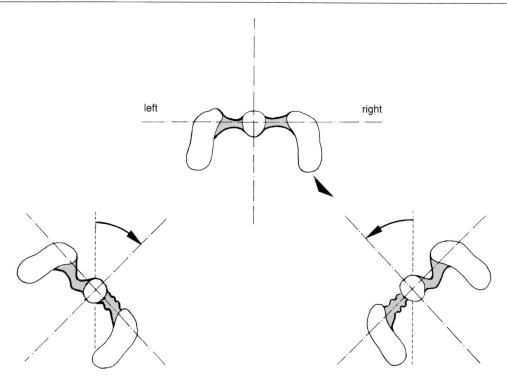

Fig. **6**. The alar ligaments during rotation of the atlantoaxial joint.

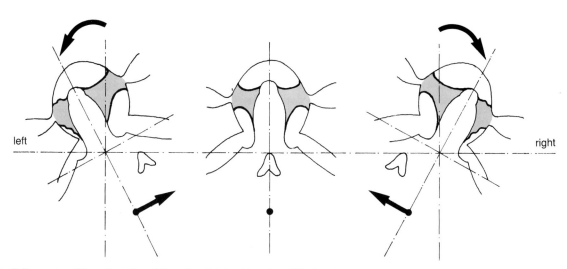

Fig. **7**. Illustration of forced rotation of the axis with lateral bending of the head.

are weak and are present inconsistently. They lead into the atlanto-occipital membrane (Fig. **8**).

Function of the Cruciform Ligament of the Atlas

The functions are to guarantee the physiological rotation of C_1–C_2 and to protect the spinal cord from the dens of the axis.

Lesions of the Alar Ligaments and the Cruciform Ligament of the Atlas

MACALISTER (1893) found that the transverse ligament of the atlas tears at a load of 130 kg. FIELDING et al. (1974) examined the tensile strength of the alar ligaments and the cruciform ligament of the atlas in 20 corpses. They found that the ligaments tear at a load of 40 to 180 kg (average, 110 kg).

The transverse ligament of the atlas tears when stretched beyond 4.8 to 7.6 mm. Overstretching will lead to tearing of the collagenous fibers, which can be seen on x-rays as an increase in the distance between the dens and the posterior surface of the anterior arch of the axis of more than 3 mm (more prominent in x-rays taken in the flexed position). With a distance of 7 mm, complete separation of the transverse ligament from the atlas is to be expected; with distances greater than 10 to 12 mm, tearing of the alar ligaments is to be expected.

The spatial relationship between the bony structures of the atlas, the dens of the axis, the spinal cord, and the free zone is designated as an anatomical constant. Generally, the rule of thirds by STEELE (1968) has proved valuable (Fig. 9). One-third of the space is occupied by the dens, one-third by the spinal cord, and one-third by a free space, the so-called safety zone of the spinal cord.

Considering the anatomical position of the cardiac and respiratory centers in the medulla oblongata, the double control is plausible in regard to the prevention of a dens dislocation via the alar ligaments and the transverse ligament of the axis. HUGUENIN (personal communication, 1980) points out the clinical symptomatology and the resulting changes seen on radiographs for the partial and complete tearing of the ligaments in the occipital-atlanto-axial joint region, both in functional and computer-directed tomograms.

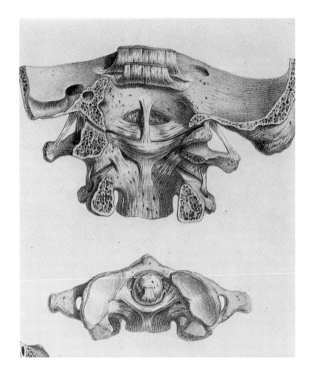

Fig. **8**. Representation of the cruciform ligament and other ligaments of the occipital-atlanto-axial complex. Above: posterior view; below: superior view (from *Arnold*, 1845).

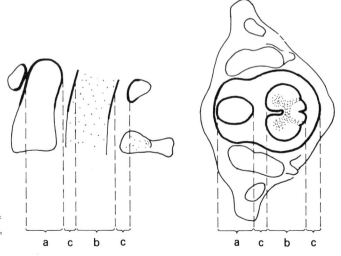

Fig. **9**. Steel's rule of thirds (1968) (schematic): a = b = 2c = ⅓ (a + b + 2c). a: dens axis; b: spinal cord, c: safety zone.

1.1.4. Functional Examination of the Occipital-Atlanto-Axial Joints

Rotation from the neutral position: This movement takes place in the entire region of the cervical spine and the first four thoracic vertebrae and measures 90° to either side (Fig. **10**).

Rotation from flexion: With maximal flexion, the lower segments of the cervical spine are locked,

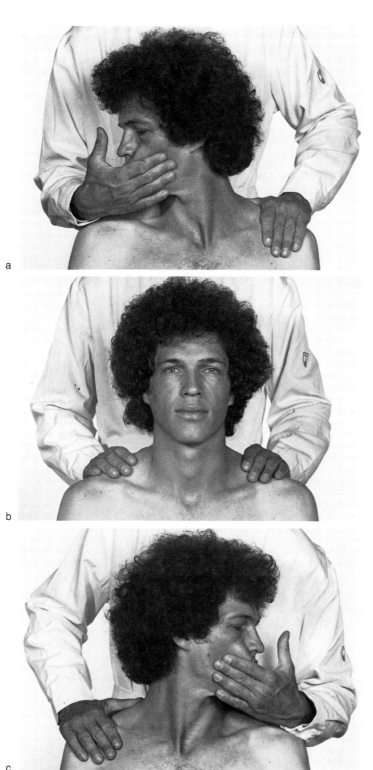

a

b

c

Fig. **10**. Rotation of the head starting from the neutral position (a: 90° to the right; b: 0°; c: 90° to the left).

that is, the individual joints are brought into their final (end) position.

Further rotation continuing from this position is then only possible in the atlantoaxial joint. Nor-mally, it measures 45° to either side (Fig. 11). A decrease in the rotation indicates a hypomobile dysfunction in the C_1–C_2 vertebral unit.

A value greater than 45° is usually the result of an

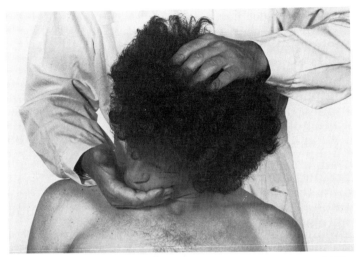

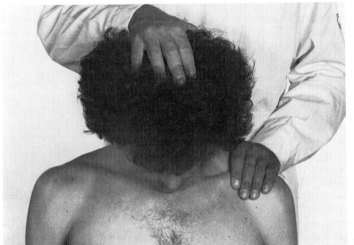

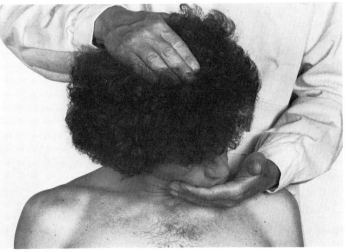

Fig. **11**. Rotation of the head starting from the flexed position (a: 45° to the right; b: 0°; c: 45° to the left).

improperly conducted examination. Seldom is it an indication of insufficient brake function of the alar ligaments (caution: hypermobility may result in a "rubberman").

Forced rotation of the axis with lateral flexion (lateralbending): The finger used for palpation rests on the spinous process of the axis while the head of the patient is laterally flexed either actively or passively. The spinous process moves simultaneously under the finger in the direction of the convexity; absence of a forced rotation therefore is to be considered pathological.

Examination of axis rotation: The biomechanics of the occipital-atlanto-axial complex shows that the rotation of the head begins in the atlantoaxial joint. It is only after the completion of this motion that the lower segments of the cervical spine begin to rotate. The rotation of the axis is palpated over the spinous process of the axis, but can be detected only after 25° to 30°. If this rotation appears earlier, it is again a sign of a hypomobile functional disorder in the occipital-atlanto-axial joints.

Palpation of the transverse process of the axis: The examiner stands behind the sitting patient. For palpation, the index finger is placed on the tip of the mastoid process and the ring finger is placed on the edge of the ramus of the mandible. The free middle finger presses deeply between these two bony projections and locates the deep transverse process of the atlas, which is normally painful upon pressure.

Terminal rotation of the atlas: Disagreement exists about the elastic rotational movement between the atlas and the occiput. According to kinematographic studies, no rotation in the atlanto-occipital joint takes place. However, when the transverse process of the axis is palpated exactly and the head rotated into its maximal position, an elastic motion of the atlas can be felt. The absense of this elastic, resilient motion, according to LEWIT (1970) and CAVIEZEL (1976), is an indication of the "blocking" (segmental dysfunction) of the atlanto-occipital-joints.

1.2.   Lower Cervical Spine

1.2.1.   Biomechanics

The axis is a transitional vertebra between the upper and lower cervical spine. The greatest range of motion takes place in the mid-cervical spine

Table **2**   Limits and Representative Values of Range of Rotation of the Lower Cervical Spine (after *White* and *Panjabi* 1978a)

Vertebral Unit	Flexion/Extension (X axis rotation)		Lateral Bending (Z axis rotation)		Axial Rotation (Y axis rotation)	
	Limits of Ranges (degrees)	Representative Angle (degrees)	Limits of Ranges (degrees)	Representative Angle (degrees)	Limits of Ranges (degrees)	Representative Angle (degrees)
C_2–C_3	5–23	8	11–20	10	6–28	9
C_3–C_4	7–38	13	9–15	11	10–28	11
C_4–C_5	8–39	12	0–16	11	10–26	12
C_5–C_6	4–34	17	0–16	8	8–34	10
C_6–C_7	1–29	16	0–17	7	6–15	9
C_7–T_1	4–17	9	0–17	4	5–13	8

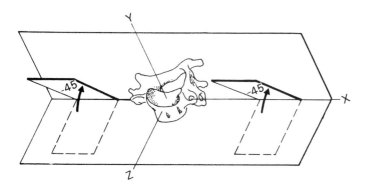

Fig. **12**. Graphical representation of the facet joint inclinations and axes of motion for vertebra C_4 (after *White* and *Panjabi*, 1978a).

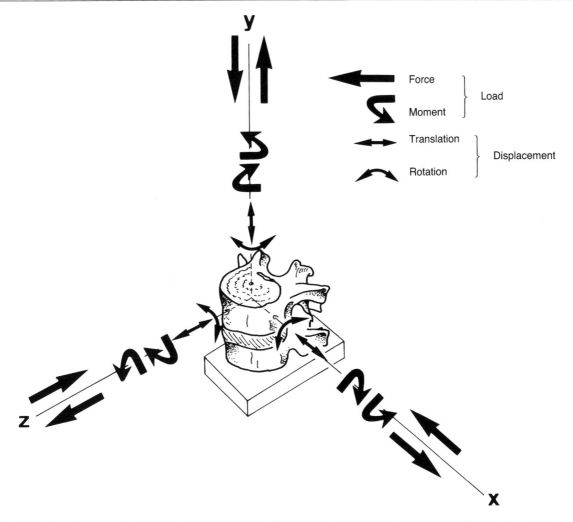

Fig. **13**. A three-dimensional coordinate system has been placed at the center of the upper vertebral body of a vertebral unit (motion segment). A total of 12 load components, linear and rotatory, can act on these axes; the application of any one of the load components (linear or rotatory) produces displacement of the upper vertebra with respect to the lower vertebra. The displacement consists of translation and rotation (after *White* and *Panjabi*, 1978a).

region where the following motions are possible: flexion/extension, lateral bending (lateral flexion), and rotation (Table **2**).

The inclination of the central and lower cervical spine facets is 45° to the horizontal plane. The lower segments are steeper than the upper segments (Fig. **12**).

The motions possible in an individual segment (vertebral unit) can be considered as the combined translatory-rotatory motion about the respective axis of the three-dimensional coordinate system (LYSELL, 1969). Rotation about the X axis is identical with flexion and extension, about the Y axis with rotation, and about the Z axis with lateral-bending (Fig. **13**).

For flexion and extension, LYSELL (1969) describes a so-called top angle up on which the individual segments move. This so-called segmental arch is flat at C_1, and almost semicircular at C_7 (Fig. **14**). The top angle is determined by the inclination of the individual facets and the condition of the intervertebral disk.

Coupling Patterns With Lateral Flexion (Lateral Bending) and Rotation

LYSELL (1969) postulated and measured the coupling patterns for lateral flexion and rotation of the cervical spine. These coupling patterns are of clinical importance and are evaluated during the functional examination.

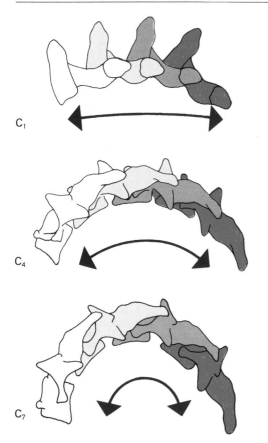

Fig. **14**. Diagrammatic representation of the segmental arches after *Lysell* (1969) (from *White* and *Panjabi*, 1978 b).

When the head is laterally flexed, the spinous processes move in the direction of the convexity, that is, in lateral bending to the left they move to the right. Motion about the Z axis is coupled to a rotation about the Y axis, and vice versa. At the second cervical vertebra, there are 2° of coupled axial rotation for every 3° of lateral bending. At the seventh cervical vertebra, there is 1° of coupled rotation for every 7.5° of lateral bending (WHITE and PANJABI, 1978 b) (Fig. **15**).

1.2.2. Functional Examination of the Lower Cervical Spine

Rotation from extension: The patient sits on a stool with his thoracic spine as straight as possible. The patient's head is held with both hands in the parietal region and is extended passively. By this procedure the occipital-atlanto-axial joint is close to its barrier. This passively performed rotation of the head, coupled to slight lateral bending of the cervical spine, is now possible in the lower segments of the cervical spine only (Fig. **16**). The empirical value is listed as 60° (CAVIEZEL, 1976; LEWIT, 1970).

Rotation of the head, palpation of the spinous processes: Again, the examination is performed with the patient sitting with his thoracic spine as

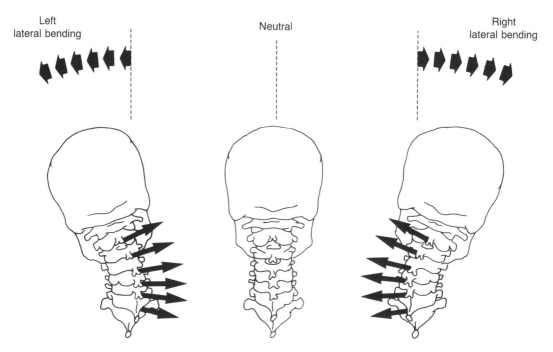

Fig. **15**. Major cervical spine coupling patterns (after *White* and *Panjabi*, 1978 b).

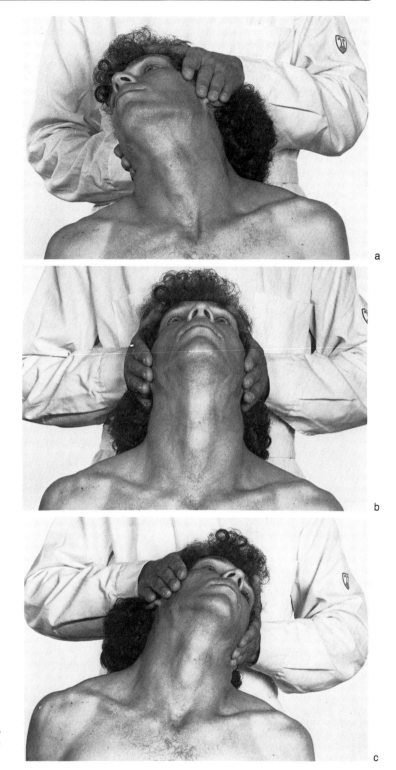

Fig. **16**. Rotation of the head starting from the extended position (a: 60° to the right; b: 0°; c: 60° to the left).

straight as possible. For palpation, the four fingers of the hand are positioned over the spinous processes of the cervical spine. The free hand guides a passive rotation of the head to both sides. Palpation with the fingers follows the range of motion of the individual spinous processes. Since the rotation (about the Y axis) at each individual segmental level is possible only to a small extent (Table **3**), the path of the individual spinous processes in the direction of the rotation is consequently very small.

Coupling patterns with lateralbending: Palpation begins with a finger resting on the spinous process while the free hand performs passive lateral flexion of the head. During lateral bending, the spinous processes move under the fingers in the direction of the convexity.

The coupling patterns, and thus the range of motion of the spinous processes, are larger in the upper segments than in the lower segments.

1.2.3. Vertebral Artery

The vertebral artery must be mentioned in connection with the functional examination and biomechanics of the cervical spine. It enters the costotransverse foramen of C_6, occasionally that of C_5, and runs to the axis through the costovertebral foramina of the individual vertebra. After a slight posterolateral curvature, it enters the costotransverse foramen of the atlas and upon exit forms a posterosuperiorly directed loop that punctures the atlanto-occipital membrane and the dura mater in the region of the foramen magnum at the occiput (Fig. **17**).

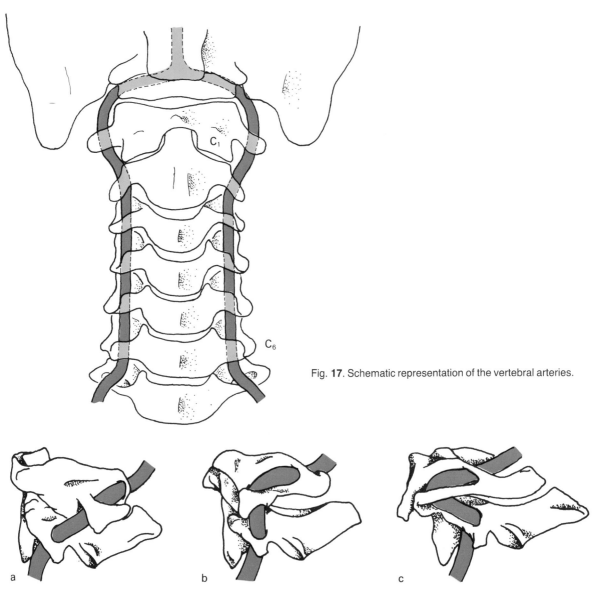

Fig. **17**. Schematic representation of the vertebral arteries.

a   b   c

Fig. **18**. Excursion of the left vertebral artery during atlas rotation to the left and to the right (after *Fielding*, 1957).

It is known that extreme rotation of the head can cause neurological symptoms, such as dizziness, nausea, and tinnitus. These are often caused by a transient, decreased blood supply in the basilar region, since rotation of the head between 30° and 45° to one side causes the blood flow to be diminished in the opposite vertebral artery at the atlantoaxial junction (FIELDING, 1957) (Fig. **18**).

It is known that "high velocity thrust techniques" can cause vascular accidents (DVORAK and ORELLI, 1982). In order to prevent accidents, it is necessary to employ provocative examination before thrust is applied (Memorandum of the German Society for Manual Medicine, 1979). It is sometimes necessary to include ultrasound examination of the vertebral artery.

Provocative test (extension and rotation of head): With the patient sitting the examiner conducts passive motion of the head to either side, starting from both the neutral and extended positions. The

passive motions should be conducted slowly, and the patient is asked to report any subjective symptom.

Kleijn Hanging Test: The patient is supine with the head beyond the examining table, being held by the examiner. From this hanging position the head is passively rotated to both sides. While the examiner observes the patient's eye movements (nystagmus), the patient is again asked to report subjective symptoms.

Ultrasound Examination: Noninvasive ultrasound examination of the carotid and vertebral arteries can be helpful when vertebral basilar insufficiency is suspected, with subclavian steal syndrome, with hypersensitive carotid sinus syndrome, and with possible increased risk of cerebral vascular disease. The ultrasound examination provides further information about the vertebral artery and its function in cervical spine motion. With an ultrasound probe of approximately 15 cm length,

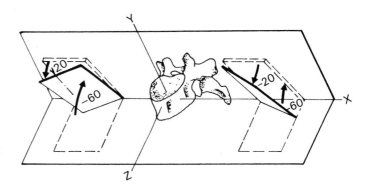

Fig. **19**. Graphical representation of the facet joint inclinations and axes of motion of a thoracic vertebra (after *White* and *Panjabi*, 1978a).

Table **3**   Limits and Representative Values of Range of Rotation of the Thoracic Spine (after *White* and *Panjabi* 1978a)

Vertebral Unit	Flexion/Extension		Lateral Bending		Axial Rotation	
	Limits of Ranges (degrees)	Representative Angle (degrees)	Limits of Ranges (degrees)	Representative Angle (degrees)	Limits of Ranges (degrees)	Representative Angle (degrees)
T_1–T_2	3–5	4	5	6	14	9
T_2–T_3	3–5	4	5–7	6	4–12	8
T_3–T_4	2–5	4	3–7	6	5–11	8
T_4–T_5	2–5	4	5–6	6	4–11	8
T_5–T_6	3–5	4	5–6	6	5–11	8
T_6–T_7	2–7	5	6	6	4–11	8
T_7–T_8	3–8	6	3–8	6	4–11	8
T_8–T_9	3–8	6	4–7	6	6–7	7
T_9–T_{10}	3–8	6	4–7	6	3–5	4
T_{10}–T_{11}	4–14	9	3–10	7	2–3	2
T_{11}–T_{12}	6–20	12	4–13	9	2–3	2
T_{12}–L_1	6–20	12	5–10	8	2–3	2

which is inserted in the oropharynx, the vertebral arteries can be detected at the C_3–C_4 level both on the left and right sides. The following criteria are diagnostically useful: direction of blood flow, differences between both vertebral arteries (diastolic phase and pulsation amplitude), reaction of the carotid upon compression, reaction upon head rotation, flexion and extension. Since it is physiological normal for blood flow to decrease with rotation, it is important to verify early blood flow arrest in this examination (ADORJANI, personal communications, 1980; KELLER et al., 1976).

1.3. Thoracic Spine

1.3.1. Biomechanics of the Thoracic Spine

The facets of the individual vertebrae show a twofold inclination, that is, inclination about the X axis of 60° and about the Y axis of 20° (Fig. **19**).

These doubly inclined facets still allow rotation about all axes (flexion and extension, lateral bending, axial rotation) (Table **4**). Lateral bending of the thoracic spine is accompanied by axial rotation (coupling patterns; Fig. **22**). It is a well-known fact that the thoracic spine is the segment of the vertebral column with the least amount of motion. The small range of motion between the vertebrae is the result of the functional arrangement of the longitudinal ligament, the annulus fibrosus, and the position of the spinous processes.

1.3.2. Biomechanics of the Thorax and Ribs

The union of the thoracic spine with the ribs and consequently with the sternum significantly increases the rigidity and stability of the longest

portion of the vertebral column. Strong ligaments stabilize the costovertebral and costotransverse joints (Fig. **20**).

The relatively rigid union between the sternum and the thoracic spine by way of the ribs markedly increases the resistance of the spine against forces that cause rotation. An interesting experiment was conducted by SCHULZ et al. (1974a). Loads were applied to individual ribs from different directions and the mobility of the ribs was measured. It was noted that the second rib exhibited the greatest resistance when the force was applied from the posteroanterior direction. The lowest stiffness and resistance (highest flexibility) was exhibited by the tenth rib when loaded either from the superior or inferior direction. According to PANJABI et al. (1978), the costovertebral joints play an important role in the stability and the segmental mobility of the thoracic spine. Their function, in addition to the stabilizing action of the whole thorax, is verified in a mathematical model by ANDRIACCHI et al. (1974).

1.3.3. Functional Examination of Thoracic Spine and the Ribs

According to LEWIT (1977), the functional examination of the thoracic spine is best conducted with the patient sitting. The patient sits on the edge of the examination table holding the hands behind the neck.

Testing of flexion-extension: The examiner conducts passive flexion and extension by grasping the arms of the patient. Moving the patient in a specific manner and following his motion, the examiner determines the range of motion in a particular vertebral unit. The fingers of the free hand concur-

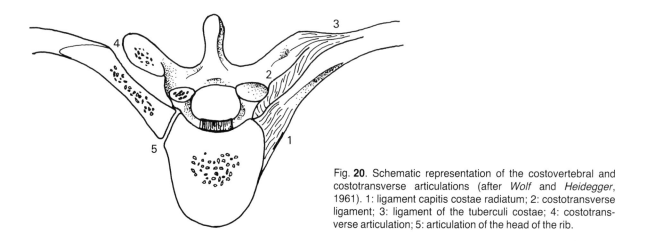

Fig. **20**. Schematic representation of the costovertebral and costotransverse articulations (after *Wolf* and *Heidegger*, 1961). 1: ligament capitis costae radiatum; 2: costotransverse ligament; 3: ligament of the tuberculi costae; 4: costotransverse articulation; 5: articulation of the head of the rib.

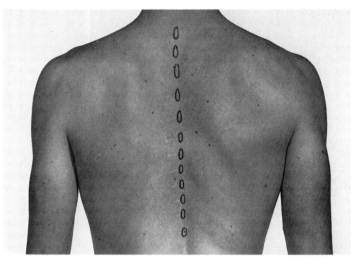

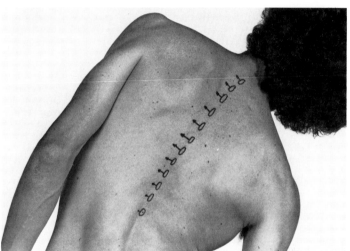

Fig. **21**. Examination of lateral bending.

rently follow the movements of the individual spinous processes.

Testing of lateral bending (coupling patterns): The patient's arms are grasped from below, the contralateral shoulder is fixed with one hand. The fingers of the free hand rest over the spinous processes. When bent laterally, the spinous processes normally move in the direction of the convexity (Fig. **21**).

Testing of rotation: The hand of the examiner is guided under the patient's axilla and grasps the opposite shoulder. After maximal rotation to one side, the arms are switched, and rotation to the other side follows (Fig. **22**). Rotation usually 60 to 80° to either side and should be strictly about the Y axis of the spine. In this examination, the range of motion of the individual spinous processes is being evaluated as well.

Testing of the ribs: The intercostal spaces are inspected and palpated both in the prone and supine position. One looks for asymmetries during the respiratory movements. With the patient sitting, the arm on the side being examined is lifted, and again the individual ribs and intercostal spaces are palpated during lateral bending. In this examination, any asymmetries will indicate hypo- or hypermobile functional disorders.

1.4.   Lumbar Spine

1.4.1.   Biomechanics of the Lumbar Spine

Motion in the region of the lumbar spine, is possible about all three axes. Motion about the X axis (flexion and extension) increases in the inferior direction, the maximum of motion being in the vertebral unit L_5–S_1 (Table **5**). Lateral bending and

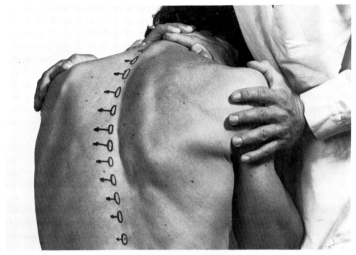

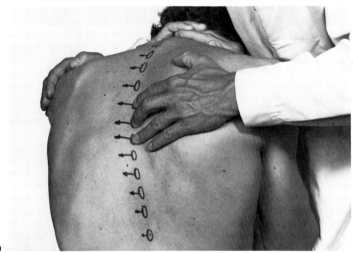

Fig. **22**. Examination of rotation.

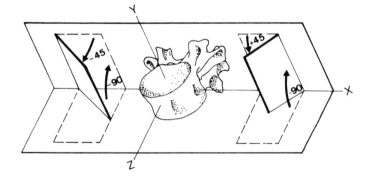

Fig. **23**. Graphical representation of the facet joint inclinations and axes of motion of a lumbar vertebra (after *White* and *Panjabi*, 1978a).

Table **4**   Representative Values of the Range of Rotation of the Lumbar Spine (after *White* and *Panjabi* 1978a)

Vertebral Unit	Flexion/Extension (X axis rotation)		Lateral Bending (Z axis rotation)		Axial Rotation (Y axis rotation)	
	Limits of Ranges (degrees)	Representative Angle (degrees)	Limits of Ranges (degrees)	Representative Angle (degrees)	Limits of Ranges (degrees)	Representative Angle (degrees)
L_1–L_2	9–16	12	3–8	6	1–3	2
L_2–L_3	11–18	14	3–9	6	1–3	2
L_3–L_4	12–18	15	5–10	8	1–3	2
L_5–S_1	14–21	17	5–7	6	1–3	2
	18–22	20	2–3	3	3–6	5

rotation about the Z axis are smallest in the lumbosacral junction. According to LUMSDEN and MORRIS (1968), axial rotation is greatest in the lumbosacral junction. Compared with lateral bending and axial rotation, flexion and extension are large, which is easily explained by the arrangement of the facets (Fig. **23**).

1.4.2. Functional Examination of the Lumbar Spine

The mobility of the individual vertebral units is examined in addition to the classic examinations, such as the determination of the fingertip-to-floor distance in the flexed position and the Schober test.

Flexion-extension: The patient lies on the side with thighs flexed 90°. The examiner locates the individual spinous processes. Subsequently, the thighs are flexed to a maximum, and the lumbar lordosis is diminished. The increased distance between the adjacent spinous processes can be felt by palpation, providing an indirect indication concerning the extent of rotation about the X axis.

Lateral bending (lateral flexion): The patient lies on the side with the legs flexed about 90° both in the hip as well as in the knee joints. The examiner grasps both legs with one hand, raising them as high as possible, which results in the lateral bending of the lumbar spine. His free hand palpates the distance and motion between the spinous processes (rotation about the Z axis).

Rotation of the L_5–S_1 vertebral unit: Rotation in the upper vertebral units of the lumbar spine is not more than 2° and can thus barely be detected. Only rotation in the lumbosacral junction (5 to 6°) can be felt by palpation.

The patient is sitting astride at the end of the examination table, while interlocking the hands behind the head. The examiner embraces the patient's trunk at shoulder level with one arm and performs a passive rotation. The index finger of the free hand rests on the upper portion of the median sacral crest while the thumb follows the motion of the spinous process of L_5. Again, rotation of the trunk increases the distance between the spinous processes, giving evidence of the mobility in the lumbosacral junction (rotation about the Y axis).

1.5.   Pelvis

1.5.1.   Biomechanics of the Pelvis

The functional unit of the pelvis consists of the sacrum, hip bones, L_5 connected through the sac-

roiliac joints (SIJ), and the symphysis pubis. Structurally, the SIJs are a diarthrosis, yet function as an amphiarthrosis due to the irregular auricular articulating surface. With increasing age, the mobility of the SIJ is further decreased through the process of ankylosis. At an age as early as the 50s, 85 percent of men and 50 percent of women show osteophytes in the SIJ. By the 60s, 60 percent of the men but only 15 percent of the women show either partial or complete ankylosis of the SIJ (FRIGERIO, 1974).

SCHMID (1980) used the roentgeno-stereophotogrammetric method developed by SELVIK (1974) to measure the mobility of the SIJ's nutation-motion. Like FRIGERIO (1974), he demonstrated mobility but of smaller extent. Both authors agree on the complexity of the SIJ motion.

SUTTER (1977) postulates four SIJ axes about which motion can take place both unilaterally and bilaterally (Fig. **24**).

The ligaments of the SIJ amphiarthrosis, in addition to the tight joint capsule, play an extremely important role. According to SUTTER (1977), the sacrum is attached to the sacroiliac ligament below the posterior projections of the iliac tuberosity. The correct position of the sacrum is not only maintained by the antagonistic action of the sacroiliac ligaments, but also by the inferior convergence and the twisted arrangement of the sacroiliac articular surfaces.

"Forces acting upon the sacrum or the hip bones are progressively resisted by the so-called 'clamp mechanism.' This mechanism functions only as long as the short sacroiliac ligaments guarantee the mechanically necessary posterior interlocking between the sacrum and both ilia. If these ligaments, however, fall short of their function, the ilia can move laterally to a very small degree. When the ilia move laterally, the upper pole of the sacrum is consequently pulled into the posterior direction by that motion and is brought closer to the protrusion of the tuberosity of the ilium. This is achieved by the fibers of the short, but strong, interosseous sacroiliac ligament" (SUTTER, 1977) (Fig. **25**).

1.5.2. Functional Examination of the Pelvis

Spine-Test: The patient stands with his back to the examiner. While the examiner places one thumb on the posterior superior iliac spine, his other thumb locates the median sacral crest at the same

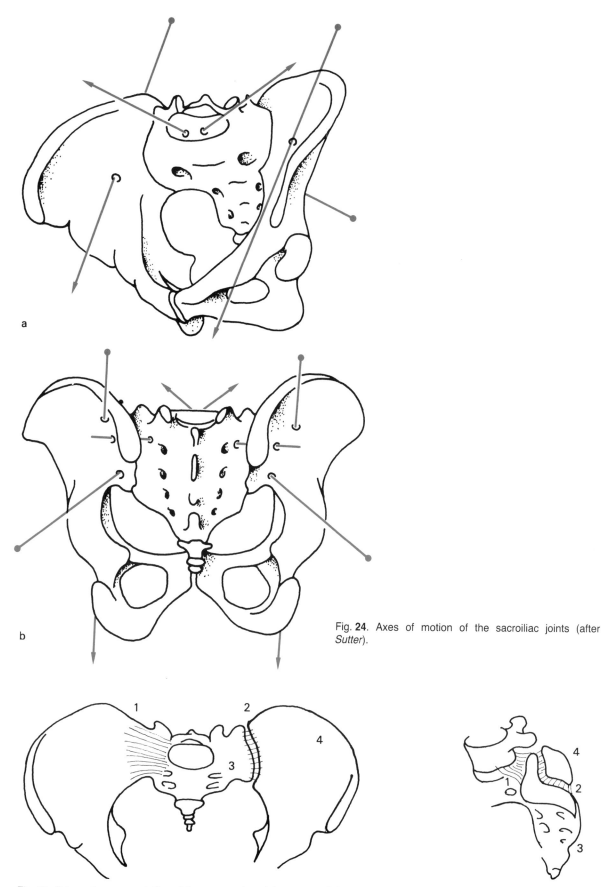

a

b

Fig. 24. Axes of motion of the sacroiliac joints (after *Sutter*).

Fig. 25. Schematic representation of the suspension of the sacrum (left: superior view; right: medial view). 1: anterior sacroiliac ligament; 2: interosseous sacroiliac ligament; 3: sacrum; 4: ilium.

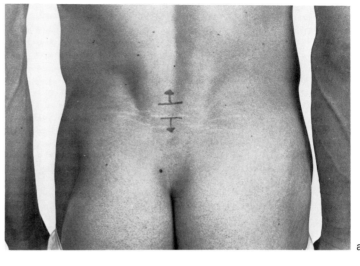

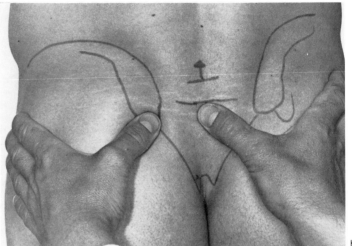

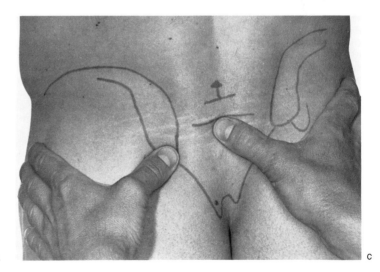

Fig. **26**. Spine test.

level. The thumbs are pressed firmly against these bony structures.

When the leg on the same side as the palpated posterior superior iliac spine is lifted, the spine moves inferiorly and laterally. If the nutation (motion in the SIJ) is absent, the spine moves superiorly due to tilting of the pelvis on the contralateral side. In this test it is important to be in very close contact with the bony structures in order during palpation to prevent the finger from sliding over the soft tissue (Fig. **26**).

Standing flexion test: Both thumbs palpate the posterior superior iliac spines from below and follow their position and motion during forward bending of the upper trunk. If the nutation motion

in the SIJ is restricted on one side, the posterior superior iliac spine is drawn superiorly with the sacrum (as compared to the opposite side) (Fig. **27**).

Uneven leg length: The leg on the side where there is no motion in the SIJ seems shorter when the patient is in a supine position, and when the patient is sitting, the leg appears to be longer.

Sign of fours, according to Kubis or Patrick: With the pelvis slightly fixed, the opposite leg is everted as far as possible. If motion in the SIJ is absent, the distance between the patella and the edge of the table is greater than that on the healthy side (caution: coxarthrosis may exist).

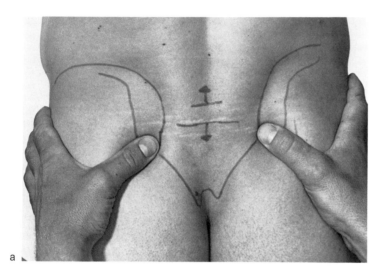

a

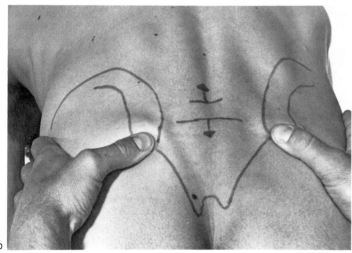

b

Fig. **27**. Standing flexion test.

2. Neuropathophysiology of the Apophyseal Joints

It is not the intention of this chapter to treat the different theories and hypotheses developed in relation to manual medicine. Little is actually known about those neurophysiological processes that are initiated with manipulation or mobilization of the apophyseal joints and joints of the extremities.

In light of the increased interest in manual medicine among physicians, it became necessary to support and promote clinical and basic research. An important step was undertaken in 1975 upon the recommendation of the National Institutes of Health. Upon the invitation of the National Institute of Neurological and Communicative Disorders and Stroke (GOLDSTEIN, 1975) a conference was held with the topic "The Research Status of Spinal Manipulative Therapy." We refer here mainly to SATO's (1975) work on the somatosympathetic reflexes, PERL's (1975) work on pain and spinal and peripheral nerve factors and WHITE and PANJABI's work (1978 b) on the biomechanics of the spine.

In 1978, a symposium was held in Pisa, Italy on "Reflex Control of Posture and Movement" (GRANIT and POMPEIANO, 1979). Even though manual medicine was not discussed per se, this symposium offers a broad basis for the theoretical research in this field.

Based on his basic experimental research with FREEMAN (1967), WYKE coined the expression "articular neurology." His work, published in 1967, 1975 (WYKE and POLACEK), 1979, and 1980, and that of JAYSON (1980) make use of this expression and help us to better understand the neurophysiological processes involved in manual medicine, to be described subsequently.

2.1. Articular Neurology

The following presentation is based mainly on the work by WYKE and coworkers.

This branch of neurology deals with the morphology, physiology, pathology, and the clinical aspects of the innervation of the joints of the whole skeleton. Here, we concentrate on the apophyseal joints.

WYKE's important contribution regarding articular neurology is the description of the structure and innervation pattern of the four receptor types, their distribution and characteristic behavior, the evidence of their presence in all synovial joint capsules, and their effects on static and dynamic reflex controls of the striated musculature, under both normal and pathological conditions.

2.1.1. Receptors of the Joint Capsule

It is well known that all synovial joints in the human body are supplied by the mechanoreceptors and nociceptive-free nerve endings (nociceptors). Their organization was visualized in neurohistological studies (WYKE and POLACEK, 1973 and 1975; FREEMAN and WYKE, 1967; VRETTOS and WYKE, 1979; Table 5).

Type-1-Receptors (Mechanoreceptors)

This type of mechanoreceptor consists of multiple, three to eight, thinly encapsulated, globular corpuscles (100 µm × 40 µm) that are found in the outer layer of the fibrous joint capsule. The thinly myelinated (6 to 9 µm) afferent nerve fibers connect these corpuscles with the corresponding articular branches of the dorsal rami of the spinal nerves.

Function:

- Slowly adapting receptors. They control tension of the outer layers of the joint capsule

- Trans-synaptic inhibition of the centripetal flow of the activity of the nociceptive afferent receptors (type IV nociceptors) or, in other words, inhibition of the impulses arising from pain receptors

- Tonic reflexogenic effects on the motoneurons ot the neck, limb, jaw, and eye muscles (WYKE, 1975, 1977; MOLINA et al., 1976; BIEMOND and DEJONG, 1969; IGARASHI et al., 1972; HIKOSAKA and MAEDA, 1973; DEJONG et al., 1977)

Table **5**   Morphological and Functional Characteristics of Articular Receptor Symptoms (*Wyke*, 1979b; *Freeman* and *Wyke*, 1967)

Type	Morphology	Location	Parent Nerve Fibers	Behavioral Characteristics	Function
I	Thinly-encapsulated globular corpuscles (100 μm × 40 μm) in clusters of 3–8	Fibrous capsulae of joint (superficial layers)	Small myelinated (6–9 μm)	Static and dynamic mechanoreceptors: low threshold, slowly adapting	Tonic reflexogenic effects on neck, limb, jaw and eye muscles. Postural and kinesthetic sensation. Pain suppression
II	Thickly encapsulated conical corpuscles (280 μm × 100 μm) singly or in clusters of 2–4	Fibrous capsulae of joint (deeper layers). Articular fat pads	Medium myelinated (9–12 μm)	Dynamic mechano-receptors: low threshold, rapidly adapting	a) Phasic reflexogenic effects on neck, limb, jaw and eye muscles. b) Pain suppression
III	Fusiform corpuscles (600 μm × 100 μm) usually singly, also in clusters of 2–3	Ligaments, also in related tendons	Large myelinated (13–17 μm)	Mechanoreceptor, high threshold, very slowly adapting	
IV	Three-dimensional plexus of unmyelinated nerve fibres	Entire thickness of fibrous capsulae of joint. Walls of articular blood vessels. Articular fat pads	Very small myelinated (2–5 μm), and unmyelinated	Nociceptive (pain-provoking). High threshold, nonadapting	a) Tonic reflexogenic effects on neck, limb, jaw and eye muscles. b) Evocation of pain. c) Respiratory and cardiovascular reflexogenic effects

Type II Receptors (Mechanoreceptors)

The type II receptors consist of oblong, conical, thickly encapsulated corpuscles (about 280 μm × 100 μm) that appear most often singly in the deeper layers of the fibrous joint capsule. These receptors are connected with the articular rami by way of the thickly myelinated nerve fibers.

Function:

- Rapidly adapting mechanoreceptors with a low threshold reacting to changes in tension of the fibrous joint capsule (less than 0.5 seconds)
- Phasic and reflexogenic effects on neck, limb, jaw, and eye muscles
- Transitory inhibition of the nociceptive activity of the joint capsule

Type III Receptors (Mechanoreceptors)

Mechanoreceptors of the type III category are the typical receptors of the ligaments and tendons inserting close to the joint capsule and are not found in the joint capsule itself. They do, however, play an important role in relation to the function of the joint. Morphologically, they consist of broad, fusiform corpuscles (600 μm × 100 μm) and usually appear singly. Occasionally, they occur in clusters of one to three and are found at the end of the ligament or tendon.

Type III receptors are innervated by large myelinated (13 to 17 μm) fibers and are connected with the articular branches. Their form resembles the ligamentous receptors of the Golgi's corpuscles, and one assumes that they have the same function. Furthermore it is believed that these slowly adapting receptors have an inhibitory reflexogenic effect on motoneurons (FREEMAN and WYKE, 1967).

Type IV Receptors (Nociceptors)

Nociceptive fibers are sensitive to noxious changes in the tissue. The nociceptors are free, very thinly myelinated or nonmyelinated plexiform nerve endings. They are ubiquitous in the fibrous portion of the joint capsule. This receptor system is activated by depolarization of the nerve fibers. For instance, depolarization occurs with constant pressure on the joint capsule (such as nonphysiological position and abrupt motions), with narrowing of the intervertebral disk, with fracture of the vertebral body, with dislocation of the apophyseal joints, or with chemical irritation (for example, potassium ions, lactic acid, 5-hydroxytryptamine, and histamine), as well as with interstitial edema of the joint capsule in acute or chronic inflammatory processes.

Function:

- Tonic reflexogenic effects on neck, limb, jaw, and eye muscles
- Evocation of pain
- Respiratory and cardiovascular reflexogenic effects

2.1.2. Innervation of the Joint Capsule

The joint capsules are supplied by the dorsal rami of the spinal nerves. It should be emphasized that the articular rami of a nerve root are not only contributing to one segmental joint capsule, but that collateral rami lead to neighboring joints as

well. Therefore the joint capsules are innervated pluri-segmentally. The cross-section of the thoracic spine, for instance, shows the nerve supply of the joints, tendons, paravertebral musculature, and the periosteum (Fig. **28**).

2.1.3. Central Interaction of the Mechanoreceptors and Nociceptor Impulses

Figure **29** shows in a simplified manner that the nociceptive and mechanoreceptive fibers enter the gray matter of the spinal cord through the dorsal root in the posterior horn. In the spinal cord the nociceptive fibers divide into many collateral rami. Some of these rami run through the gray matter directly to the basal nuclei (basal spinal nucleus or lamina IV and V after Rexed). Furthermore, they run through the lateral spinothalamic tract (anterolateral) and reach the limbic system, where the actual perception of pain occurs. Pain cannot

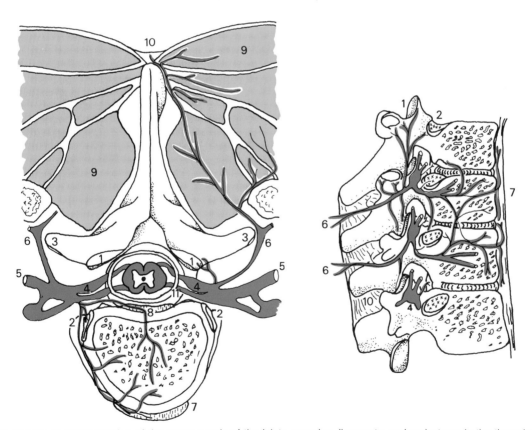

Fig. **28**. Schematic representation of the nerve supply of the joints, muscles, ligaments, and periosteum in the thoracic spine region: 1: Apophyseal joint; 2: costovertebral joint; 3: costotransverse joint; 4: spinal ganglion; 5: ventral ramus of the spinal nerve; 6: dorsal ramus of the spinal nerve; 7: anterior longitudinal ligament; 8: posterior longitudinal ligament; 9: paravertebral musculature; 10: interspinous ligament; 11: ventral ramus of the spinal nerve (after *Wyke*, 1967).

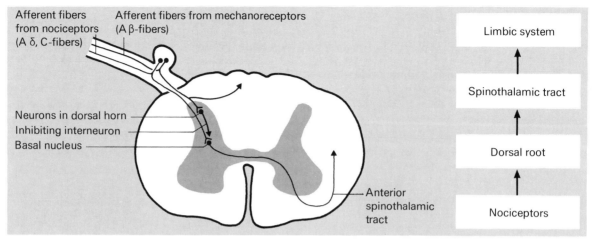

Fig. **29**. Fibers of nociceptors and mechanoreceptors in the region of the posterior horns (after *Wyke*, 1979 a).

be subjectively perceived unless depolarization of the synapse has occurred at the level of the basal nuclei as a result of the nociceptive impulses.

The mechanoreceptive afferent fibers enter the posterior horn of the gray matter of the spinal cord through the dorsal root (Fig. **29**). Important for our theory is the fact that some of the many divided rami form synapses at the level of the apical spinal nucleus (or lamina II after Rexed). The apical spinal interneurons arising from this location conduct the activity of the mechanoreceptive afferent stimuli to the basal spinal nucleus and, at this level, are thus able to presynaptically inhibit the arriving pain-inducing nociceptor stimuli to a certain extent. Thus, they interrupt conduction to the spinothalamic tract and the limbic system (Wyke, 1979; Bonica and Albe-Fessard, 1980).

2.1.4. Mechanoreceptors and Nociceptive Reflexes

A significant contribution to the understanding and the basis for research of the clinically observed spondylogenic reflex syndrome (SRS) came from Wyke and coworkers. This experimental work is of such significance that it is described here in detail.

In anesthestized cats, the joint capsule and the articular nerve C_3–C_4 were microsurgically exposed. Using a probe and a stimulator, the joint capsule was irritated. To stimulate the mechanoreceptors, a substantially lower voltage (2 V) was necessary than for the stimulation of the nociceptors (8 V). Wyke's results, reproduced here, show very clearly the reflexogenic relation-

ship between the receptors of the fibrous joint capsule, the apophyseal joints, and the peripheral musculature (Figs. **30, 31, 32, 33**).

Sato (1975) made similar observations in his investigation of the somatosympathetic reflexes. Perl (1975) views this mechanism as a partial explanation of the so-called referred pain. Wyke (1979b) suspects multisynaptic intraspinal tracts, both ascending to the brainstem and descending to the basal nuclei of the lower levels of the spinal cord.

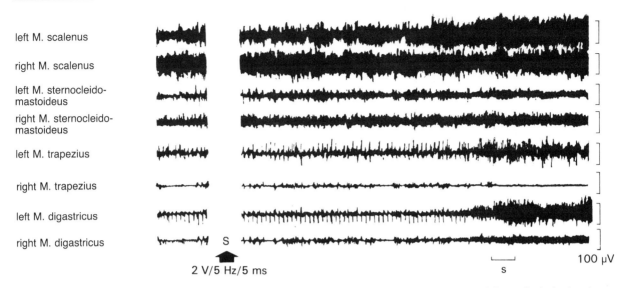

Fig. **30**. The reflexogenic mechanoreceptor effects of a cervical apophyseal joint on the musculature of the neck. At the location indicated by the arrow (S) a single articular nerve of the left C_3–C_4 apophyseal joint was stimulated for 3 seconds with an electrical impulse (2 v, 5 Hz, 5 ms) that selectively excited the mechanoreceptive afferent fibers in the exposed nerve. The simultaneous electromyographic tracings show a long-lasting effect on the homologous pairs of the neck musculature (after *Wyke*, 1979).

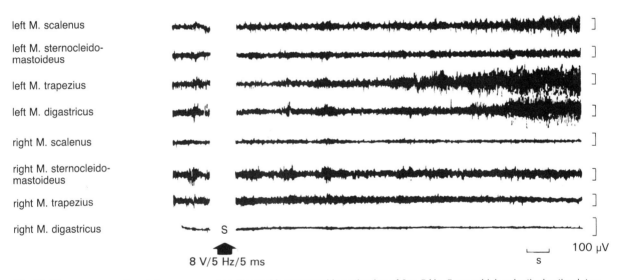

Fig. **31**. The same experimental arrangement as Figure **30**, except with a stimulus of 8 v, 5 Hz, 5 ms, which selectively stimulates not only the mechanoreceptive, but also the nociceptive afferent fibers (after *Wyke*, 1979).

left M. biceps brachii

left M. triceps brachii

left M. rectus femoris

left M. biceps femoris

right M. biceps brachii

right M. triceps brachii

right M. rectus femoris

right M. biceps femoris

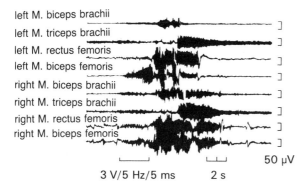

3 V/5 Hz/5 ms   2 s   50 µV

Fig. **32**. Reflex effects of the mechanoreceptors of the cervical apophyseal joints on limb muscles. At the signal (S), a single, exposed ramus of the articular nerve was repetitively stimulated for 3 seconds exciting selectively the mechanoreceptor afferent fibers in the corresponding nerve. The simultaneous electromyographic tracings of the upper and lower limb muscles display the reflexogenic effects of varying duration and indicate that such inputs affect not only the limb muscles but also the neck muscles (see Fig. **30**). It is interesting to note that the stimulation with a nociceptive impulse produces a different muscle potential response (after *Wyke*, 1979).

left M. biceps brachii

left M. triceps brachii

left M. rectus femoris

left M. biceps femoris

right M. biceps brachii

right M. triceps brachii

right M. rectus femoris

right M. biceps femoris

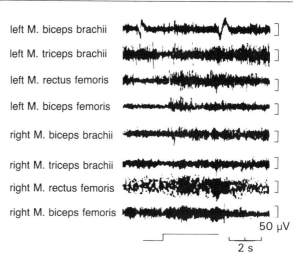

50 µV

2 s

Fig. **33**. The reflex effects of articular manipulation at C_3–C_4. At the signal, a rapid vertical traction procedure was applied across the isolated joint. The simultaneous electromyographic tracings of the homologous pairs of the upper and lower limb muscles display the reflex effects of such cervical manipulation on the peripheral musculature (after *Wyke*, 1979).

3. Differential Diagnosis and Definition of the Radicular and Spondylogenic (Nonradicular) Pain Syndromes

In 1955 GUTZEIT identified two important historical starting points documenting the importance of the vertebral factors in the clinical presentation:

- The operation of the herniated intervertebral disk by MIXTER and BARR in 1934 by which the "rheumatic" ischialgia could be healed
- The perception by osteopathic physicians and chiropractors that pain caused by the vertebrae can be influenced through manual treatment of the spine

Both points are still of great significance. Diagnosis of the objective radicular failure, clarification through radiology (myelography and computer tomography [CT] scan, including three-dimensional reconstructive recordings [GLEN et al., 1979]), as well as precise palpatory examination of the spine and the paraspinal soft tissue are all prerequisites to allow a clear decision as to what procedure is to be applied: either the surgical removal of a radicular compression syndrome, be it the result of a herniated intervertebral disk or bony new growth, or the manual treatment of the spine when a spondylogenic (nonradicular) pain syndrome is present.

As a result of their extensive palpatory experience, manual therapists (MAIGNE, 1970; LEWITT, 1977), osteopathic physicians (JONES, 1981; MITCHELL et al., 1979), and chiropractors (WALTHER, 1981) have made considerable contributions in the field of functional diagnosis of the musculoskeletal system, especially the vertebral column and the paraspinal tissue.

For patients with an acute radicular syndrome, there is little diagnostic difficulty, which is not the case for patients with chronic back pain, some differentiation for further therapy is especially important, although not always simple. One often finds a mixed clinical picture, adding to the difficulty of diagnosis. When testing for the radicular syndrome, particular attention is to be paid to the motor disturbances and the deep tendon reflexes. When examining sensory radicular disorders, the attention should be directed toward the algesias.

The hypoesthesias (decreased touch perception) and paresthesias (abnormal perception; tickling to numbness) are only of limited value, since these symptoms are typical of nonradicular syndromes (BRÜGGER, 1977; FEINSTEIN et al., 1954; KELLGREN 1939).

For the classic neurological examination procedure of the root syndromes, one should consult the pertinent textbooks.

3.1. Radicular Syndromes

3.1.1. Anatomy of the Spinal Nerves

All but three of the 31 pairs of nerve roots exit the spinal column through the intervertebral foramina. The first cervical root exits between the atlas and the occiput, and the last sacral and the only coccygeal nerve exit via the sacral hiatus (Fig. **34**).

The faster growth rate of the vertebral column results in a height difference between the spinal cord level and the vertebral level. Due to this displacement, the nerve roots in the lumbar and sacral region run laterally and almost vertically to their point of exit in the intervertebral foramen. This is in contrast to the cervical roots, which are mostly horizontal. The length of the roots increases from a few millimeters to about 25 cm (MUMENTHALER and SCHLIACK, 1982).

The spinal cord inferior to L_2 contains nerve roots only, commonly called the cauda equina.

The spinal nerve roots are positioned for the most part intradurally. The pia mater covers the beginning portions, and the arachnoid runs along the roots, terminating at the root pockets formed by the dura. Both the anterior and the posterior roots exit through separate openings in the dura before they unite to form the spinal nerves. After leaving the intervertebral foramen, the spinal nerve divides into four typical rami (Fig. **35**).

The meningeal nerve, which is both sensory and autonomic, returns to the spinal cord. The white

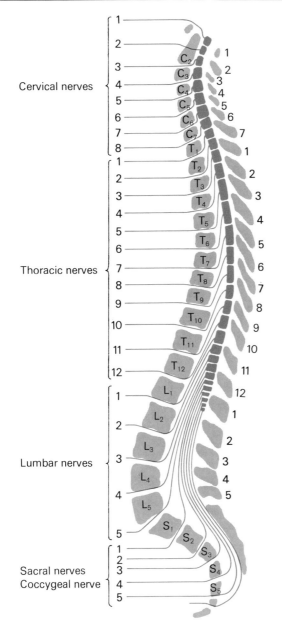

Cervical nerves

Thoracic nerves

Lumbar nerves

Sacral nerves
Coccygeal nerve

Fig. **34**. Diagram of the position of the spinal cord segments of the nerve roots with reference to the bodies and spinous processes of the vertebrae (after *Borovansky*, 1967).

and terminate at the visceral organs. Furthermore, the nerve root divides into a dorsal ramus and a ventral ramus. With the exception of the first and second dorsal rami (suboccipital nerve and greater occipital nerve, respectively), the ventral rami are substantially thicker than the dorsal rami.

Important for practical purposes is the topographical relationship of the nerve root to the intervertebral canal or the intervertebral foramen. The vertebral bodies, the vertebral arches, and the articular processes determine the bony limitations, and the joint capsule and the intervertebral disk are the soft tissue borders. Fat tissue (noted in a CT scan) and the venous plexi cushion the spinal nerve against the wall. It is of clinical significance that the diameter of the intervertebral foramina decreases from L_1 to L_5, whereas the circumference of the nerve roots increases severalfold.

In addition to radicular pain caused by compression, any of the surrounding structures (soft tissue, bones) can be a source of pain (WYKE, 1967). The joint capsule of the small apophyseal joints seems to play a special role in the nonradicular pain character or the so-called referred pain (BRÜGGER, 1977; FEINSTEIN et al., 1954; HOCKADAY and WHITTY, 1967; KELLGREN, 1938; KORR, 1975; REYNOLDS, 1981; SUTTER, 1975; WYKE, 1967 and 1979b).

3.1.2. Important Radicular Syndromes

The topographic arrangement of the nerve roots, the intervertebral canal, and disk, as well as the differing loads on the individual vertebral units, is primarily responsible for lower lumbar and first sacral nerve root compressions, as is often seen with protrusion or prolapse of the intervertebral disk. The relationship between the diameter of the nerve root and the intervertebral canal is significantly unfavorable in the lumbosacral junction in comparison to other segments of the spinal cord.

Apart from the limited spatial arrangement, it is the quite vertical course of the nerve roots in the lumbosacral junction that can cause the next root to come into contact with the intervertebral disk as well.

The posterolaterally herniated intervertebral disk of L_4–L_5 compresses primarily the fifth lumbar nerve, whereas the disk of L_5–S_1 compresses the first sacral nerve. The nerve root leaving the intervertebral foramen in this vertebral unit can exit without compression. When the hernia of the disk

communicating branch (sympathetic fibers) is directed to the corresponding ganglion of the sympathetic trunk in the paravertebral region. A section of the postganglionic, less myelinated sympathic fibers returns to the nerve roots as the gray communicating branch. The remaining fibers continue to the visceral organs. The rami communicantes contain sensory fibers in addition to autonomic fibers that pass through the ganglion

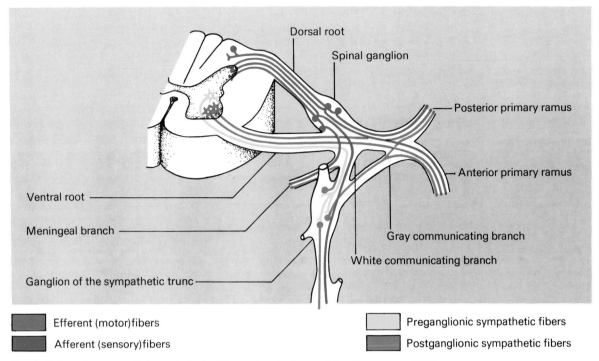

Fig. **35**. Schematic representation of individual fibers of a spinal nerve (after *Borovansky*, 1967).

is substantial, a combined L_4–L_5 and L_5–S_1 or a radicular syndrome can arise (Fig. **36**).

The occurrence of the radicular syndrome from cervical nerve roots is about 0.01 that in the lumbar region. The root of C_6 is involved most frequently due to the great mobility of the segment C_5–C_6. The thoracic root syndromes are extremely rare. The clinical presentation of a herniated disk in the center of the thoracic spine, however, can be very dramatic, since the diameter of the canal of the spinal column between T_4 and T_9 is quite small, and the vascular supply is markedly decreased in comparison to the remaining segments of the spinal cord (WHITE and PANJABI, 1978).

These two factors can result in the increased likelihood of injury as the consequence of a "contrecoup" mechanism involving the spinal cord and the nerve roots (Fig. **37**).

3.1.3. Symptomatology of the Root Syndromes

Compression of the individual nerve roots is normally accompanied by the following symptoms (Table **6**):

– Pain in the region supplied by the nerve roots

– Radicular loss of sensitivity according to the dermatomes

– Motor loss of the muscles innervated by the corresponding roots

– Deep tendon reflex disturbances

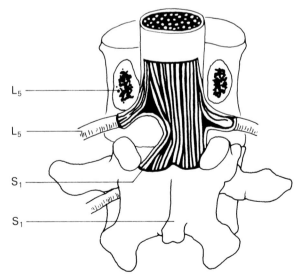

Fig. **36**. A large laterally herniated disk in the lumbosacral junction compresses upon both the first sacral and the fifth lumbar root (*Dubs*, 1950).

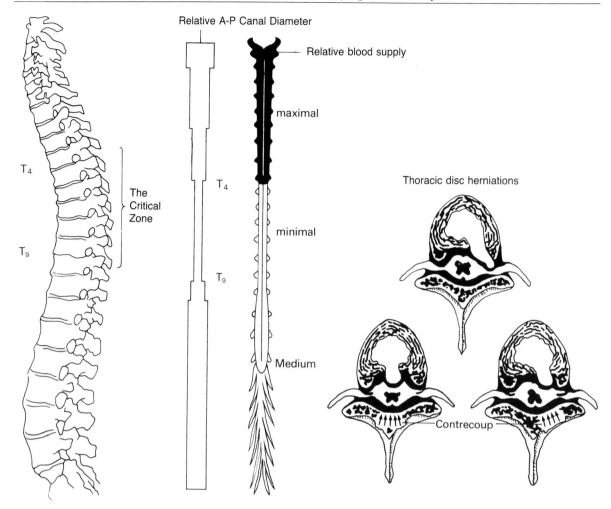

Fig. 37. Schematic representation of the cross-section of the central canal of the spinal cord and its relative blood supply. The contrecoup phenomenon for thoracic herniated disks. The relatively small cross-section and the minimal blood supply in the thoracic spine between T_4 and T_9 are responsible for the catastrophic nature of thoracic disk disease (after *White* and *Panjabi*, 1978b).

3.2.   Spondylogenic (Nonradicular) Syndrome

The observations of the nonradicular pain syndromes, to date empirical only, have been gaining more importance through the experimental neurophysiological work by KORR (1975) SIMONS (1976), and WYKE (1967 and 1979b). Different authors attempted to organize and categorize the painful soft tissue changes (often described as inflammatory soft tissue rheumatism) and furthermore to correlate them with the functional disturbances of the spinal cord or the peripheral joints (BRÜGGER, 1962, 1977; FEINSTEIN et al., 1954; HOHERMUTH, 1981; JONES, 1981; MITCHELL et al., 1979; SUTTER, 1975; SUTTER and FRÖHLICH, 1981; WALLER, 1975). The ultimate goal is to assure clear diagnostic differentiation from the actual radicular syndromes and consequently to specify the appropriate therapy, be it manipulation of the joints or stretching and rehabilitation of the muscles.

Even though the same somatic phenomena are described, the language and terminology used by the different authors reflect the individual's opinion and school of thought. The diversity of terminology and neurophysiological theories – understandable from a historical viewpoint (DVORAK, 1982; GIBSON, 1980; WARDWELL, 1980) – led to the result that these valuable clinical observations have found only limited diagnostic utilization in the mainstream of medicine.

In the following chapter, five concepts of the spondylogenic syndrome are presented. Despite

Table **6**   Review of Root Syndromes (after *Mumenthaler* and *Schliack* 1982)

Segment	Sensation	Muscles Involved	Tendon Reflex	Remarks
$C_{3/4}$	Pain (hypalgesia) in shoulder region (see Fig. **1**)	Partial or total paralysis of diaphragm	No detectable changes	Partial diaphragmatic paralysis, C_3 more ventral and C_4 more dorsal
C_5	Pain (hypalgesia) over lateral aspect of shoulder, covering deltoid area	Disturbance of innervation of deltoid and biceps brachii muscles	Diminished or absent biceps reflex	
C_6	Dermatome on outer aspect of arm and forearm as far as the thumb	Paralysis of biceps brachii and brachioradialis muscles	Diminished or absent biceps reflex	
C_7	Dermatome lateral and dorsal to C_6 dermatome, including index to ring fingers	Paralysis of triceps brachii, pronator teres and occasionally the finger flexors; often visible atrophy of the thenar eminence	Diminished or absent triceps reflex	Differential diagnosis of carpal tunnel syndrome: note the triceps reflex
C_8	Dermatome to C_7, extending to include little finger	Small muscles of hand, visible atrophy especially of hypothenar eminence	Diminished triceps reflex	Differential diagnosis of ulnar nerve palsy: note the triceps reflex
L_3	Dermatome extending from greater trochanter over the extensor surface to the medial side of the thigh and knee	Paralysis of quadriceps femoris muscle	Absent quadriceps reflex (knee jerk)	Differential diagnosis of femoral nerve palsy: area of saphenous nerve innervation remains intact
L_4	Dermatome extending from lateral surface of thigh across the knee to the anterior and medial quadrant of the leg, including the medial part of the sole	Paralysis of quadriceps femoris and tibialis anterior muscles	Diminished quadriceps reflex (knee jerk)	Differential diagnosis of femoral nerve palsy: involvement of tibialis anterior or muscle
L_5	Dermatome extending from above lateral condyle of femur, over the anterior and outer quadrant of the leg as far as the gret toe	Paralysis and atrophy of extensor hallucis longus, often also extensor digitorum brevis muscles	Absent tibialis posterior reflex, only useful if the opposite reflex can be clearly elicited	
S_1	Dermatome extending from flexor surface of thigh to outer and posterior quadrant of leg, and over the lateral malleolus to the little toe	Paralysis of peroneal muscles, frequently also disturbances of innervation of the triceps surae muscle	Absent triceps surae reflex (ankle jerk)	
Combined $L_{4/5}$	L_4 and L_5 dermatomes	All extensor muscles of ankle; also disturbances of innervation of quadriceps femoris	Diminished quadriceps reflex. Absent tibialis posterior reflex	Differential diagnosis of peroneal nerve palsy: peroneal muscles escape. Note knee jerk and tibialis posterior
Combined L_5/S_1	L_5 and S_1 dermatomes	Extensors of toes, peroneal muscles, occasionally also disturbances of innervation of triceps surae muscles	Absent tibialis posterior and triceps surae reflex	Differential diagnosis of peroneal nerve palsy: tibialis anterior muscle escapes. Note the reflex findings

the difference in terminology, the attentive reader will not miss the similarities. In order to appreciate the phenomena of the soft tissue changes in daily practice, knowledge of the topographical anatomy and palpation of the living human being is required.

The systematics of the spondylogenic reflex syndrome, worked out by SUTTER, are described in detail. Anatomical and palpatory fundamentals of the paravertebral musculature are presented to facilitate the learning of soft tissue palpation (chapters 7 and 8).

3.2.1. Referred Pain

KELLGREN (1938), SINCLAIR et al. (1948), HOCKADAY and WHITTY (1967) demonstrated in clinical experiments that local and referred pain occurs upon mechanical or chemical stimulation of different spinal and paraspinal structures.

When injecting hypertonic sodium chloride solution into the paravertebral musculature, ligaments, and apophyseal joints, or when scratching the periosteum with a needle, local and referred pain was elicited in every instance according to the segmental innervation (KELLGREN, 1938, 1939; LEWIS and KELLGREN, 1939) (Fig. 38).

When deep structures were stimulated, a diffuse pain distant from the origin of stimulation could be observed. Stimulating structures of the thoracic spine produces pain similar to skin hypersensitivity on both the anterior and posterior side of the trunk

in a patchwork manner (Fig. 39) (HOCKADAY and WHITTY, 1967). This is in contrast to a bandlike pain encircling the body in a girdle fashion when nerve lesions are present (for instance with herpes zoster).

Upon the stimulation of structures of the lumbosacral junction, the patients perceive a deep pain in the gluteal region and in the thigh, but seldom reaching below the knee.

Palpation can detect the differences between the structures affected by referred pain (muscles, ligaments, fascia) and the surrounding tissue. Local anesthesia in these secondarily altered structures reduces the referred pain. The spontaneous local pain of the originally stimulated tissue (that is, supraspinous or interspinous ligaments) is thereby influenced very little. As local anesthesia is applied around the irritated ligament, both local and referred pain disappear (KELLGREN, 1939).

The outcome of the experimental observations is summarized by KELLGREN as follows:

"The superficial fascia of the back, the spinous processes, and the supraspinous ligaments induce local pain upon stimulation, while stimulation of the superficial portions of the interspinous ligaments and the superficial muscles result in a diffused type of pain. The deep muscles, ligaments and periosteum of the apophyseal joints as well as the joints themselves can cause referred pain according to the segmental innervation when sufficiently stimulated."

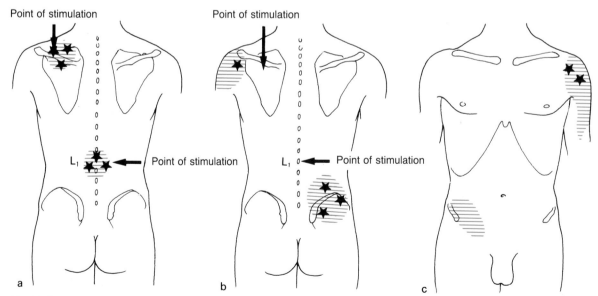

Fig. **38**. Pain pattern upon injection of hypertonic sodium chloride solution into superficial **(a)** and deep structures (vertebral arches, fossa infraspinata scapulae (after *Kellgren*, 1939).

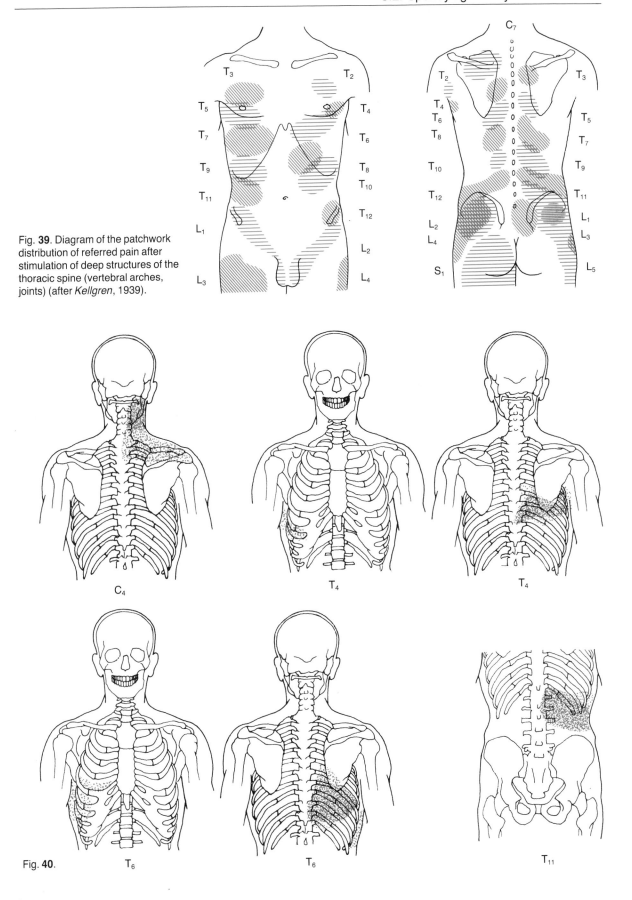

Fig. **39**. Diagram of the patchwork distribution of referred pain after stimulation of deep structures of the thoracic spine (vertebral arches, joints) (after *Kellgren*, 1939).

Fig. **40**.

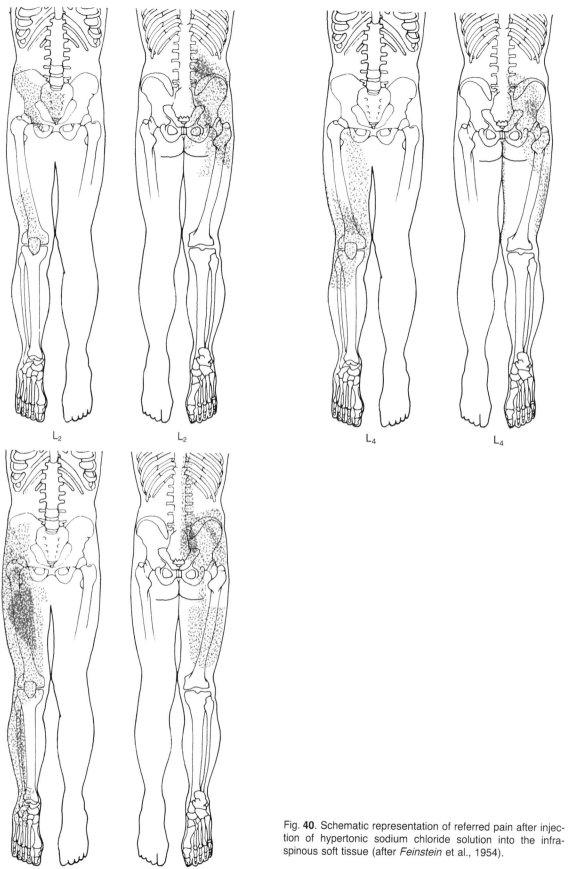

Fig. **40**. Schematic representation of referred pain after injection of hypertonic sodium chloride solution into the infraspinous soft tissue (after *Feinstein* et al., 1954).

FEINSTEIN et al. (1954) also injected a hypertonic sodium solution into the paravertebral structures of the vertebral units C_1–S_3 (deep muscles, ligaments). The manifestation of referred pain and the localization of zones with decreased sensitivity to pain did not always correlate with the radicular supply (Head zones).

Upon injection of the sodium solution pain was mostly felt in the reflexogenic hypertonic muscles and was accompanied by autonomic symptoms, such as paleness, excessive sweating, decreased blood pressure, fainting, and nausea.

Figure **40** depicts patterns of referred pain when the segments C_4, T_4, T_6, T_{11}, L_2, L_4, L_5 are stimulated.

3.2.2. Myofascial Trigger Point Syndromes

As a result of research over many decades, the myofascial trigger point, TP, has been reported by several investigators (MELZACK, 1978; REYNOLDS, 1981; RUBIN, 1981; SIMONS 1975/1976; TRAVELL and RINZLER, 1952; TRAVELL, 1976).

These points are painful either spontaneously or upon pressure and can cause referred pain in the muscles. The painful response is consistently observed in that musculature that is correlated with the TP (Fig. **41**).

The anatomical substrate (analogous to the zones of irritation) of the trigger points and the neurophysiological interaction with the referred pain in the muscles are unknown.

3.2.2.1. Trigger Points

The TP is a small (0.5 to 1 cm) area of muscle that is hypersensitive to pressure and is noticeably different from the surrounding region when palpated. The active TP has a low threshhold for mechanical stimulation. With normal physiological motion, local pain appears, but it is the referred pain in the reference musculature that is perceived by the patient as being more irritating.

The clinically asymptomatic, latent TP refers pain only when considerable palpatory pressure is applied or when an acupuncture needle is inserted into the TP (MELZACK, 1981). Characteristics of a muscle with a TP are weakness of contraction but no atrophy. Contraction leads to decreased motility of the corresponding joint (TRAVELL, 1981).

In normal muscle, a TP cannot be demonstrated and pain cannot be initiated with normal palpatory pressure.

Even though little is known about the etiology of the TP, the list of main causes includes direct muscle or joint injury, chronic muscle overload, or lengthy periods of hypothermia (TRAVELL, 1981). Latent TPs can be activated by small impulses, such as the overstretching of muscle, momentary overload, or immobilization. The formation of TPs in the segmental musculature is also known to occur with compression of the nerve root (TRAVELL, 1976). As a rule, they are not reversible, even after successful operative management (caution: postlaminectomy syndrome) (TRAVELL, 1976).

Reports exist that hypomobility of the joints, due to segmental dysfunction or inflammatory processes, can influence the development of a TP of the muscle.

3.2.2.2. Referred Pain in the Reference Site

The referred pain with active or latent TP is always localized by the patient precisely.

Using palpation, the painful muscle or part of the muscle (myotenone) can be demarcated. It is described as a "palpable band" (SIMONS, 1975/1976) which should be palpated perpendicular to the direction of the fibers (similar to the myotendinoses). Palpation often causes a local, painful twitch response in the muscle involved (SIMONS, 1976; TRAVELL and RINZLER, 1952).

One TP can cause pain in one or in several reference sites (Fig. **41**).

The induction of several so-called satellite (TPs by a primary TP is described by TRAVELL (1981). For instance, a TP in the sternal region of the sternocleidomastoid muscle can cause a satellite TP in the sternalis muscle, pectoral muscle and the serratus anterior major muscle.

In addition to causing referred pain, the active TP can influence autonomic functions in the reference site (cooling by local vasoconstriction, increased sweat secretion, increased pilomotor activity).

Occasionally, hyperalgesic skin regions can be observed (TRAVELL, 1981).

3.2.2.3. Treatment

The activity of the TP can be reduced through maximal stretching of the involved muscles. The "spray-and-stretch" method has proved to be valu-

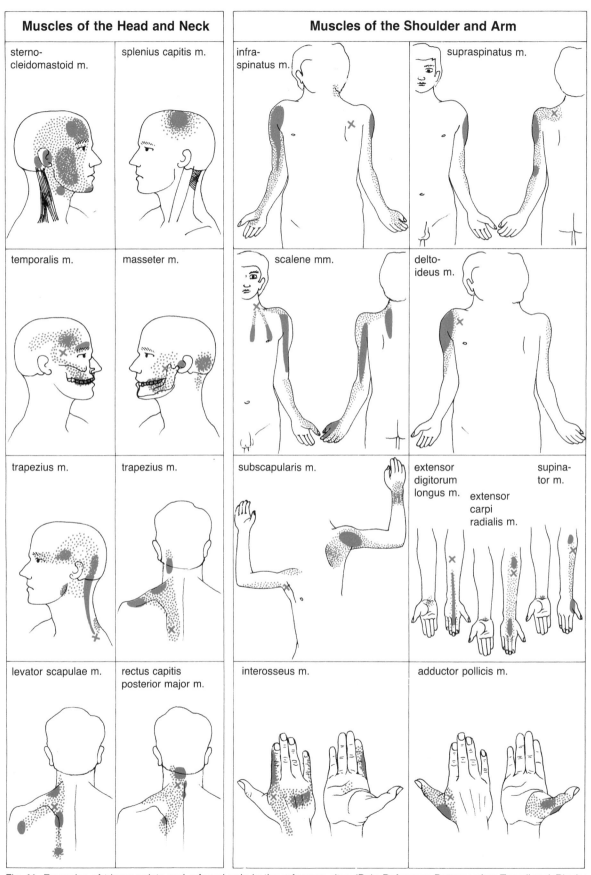

Fig. **41**. Examples of trigger points and referred pain in the reference sites (Pain Reference Pattern; after *Travell* and *Rinzler*, 1952).

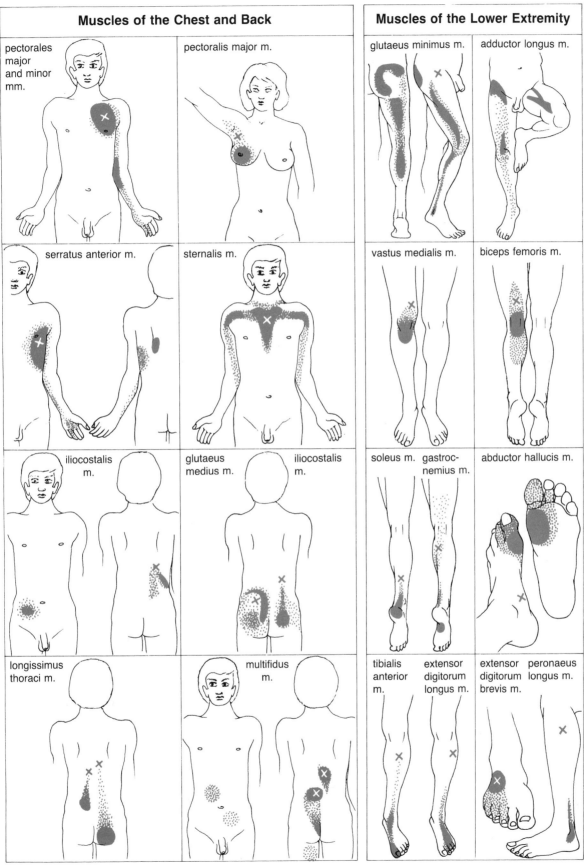

Muscles of the Chest and Back

pectorales major and minor mm.

pectoralis major m.

serratus anterior m.

sternalis m.

iliocostalis m.

glutaeus medius m.

iliocostalis m.

longissimus thoraci m.

multifidus m.

Muscles of the Lower Extremity

glutaeus minimus m.

adductor longus m.

vastus medialis m.

biceps femoris m.

soleus m.

gastrocnemius m.

abductor hallucis m.

tibialis anterior m.

extensor digitorum longus m.

extensor digitorum brevis m.

peronaeus longus m.

✘ Triggerpoint   ◼️⋮ Pain Pattern

able (TRAVELL, 1981). With the help of a cooling spray (fluorimethane), afferent nociceptive impulses of the skin are initiated. Due to the nociceptive reflexogenic influence, the shortened muscle can be stretched more easily. This stretch stimulus in turn is able to block the activity of the TP via the reflexogenic pathway through the spinal cord or possibly the higher central nervous system (CNS) center. Additionally, the TP activity can be reduced or even brought to a complete halt by injection of local anesthetics, such as procaine. The muscle involved is stretched passively during injection.

3.2.3. Pseudoradicular Syndrome

BRÜGGER (1962, 1977) makes a clear distinction between the radicular syndrome and the pseudoradicular syndrome. The pseudoradicular syndromes are based on the reflexogenic arthromuscular aspect of the disease and are the result of the nociceptive somatomotoric blocking effect (Brügger, 1977) attributable to the painfully stimulated tissues, especially the joint capsule, origins of tendons, and other soft tissue. Not only the muscles with their corresponding tendon junctions (tendomyoses) but the skin as well can be reflexogenically painful (Brügger, 1958). Tendomyosis is described as the reflexogenic functional change in the muscle in the presence of concurrent functionally dependent muscle pain. These reflexogenic reactions are initiated by nociceptor stimulation.

3.2.3.1. Sternal Syndrome

The sternal syndrome is described as the expression of the organism's reactions to the elevated sensitivity of the sternocostal and sternoclavicular region when the thoracic spine is in an abnormal or slouched position in contrast to the normal upright thorax position (Fig. **42**).

The clinical tendomyotic presentation of the sternal syndrome develops in those muscles that support the sternocostal and sternoclavicular joints (intercostal muscles, pectoralis major muscle, sternocleidomastoid muscle, scalene muscles, posterior neck muscles). The reflexogenically contracted and thus painful muscles are palpatorily examined both in the upright and in the abnormal thorax position. Tendomyoses of the pectoralis major muscle can very well imitate parasternal pain caused by organic heart diseases (Fig. **43**).

Brügger considers the effort Syndrome as a part of the sternal syndrome.

The reflexogenically hypertonic neck musculature may cause a secondary spondylogenic cervical syndrome. Sternocostal and sternoclavicular stimulation can also lead to the reflexogenic contraction of all arm muscles (myotendinosis). The clinical presentation of the reflexogenic tendomyoses is significantly different for the upright and normal thorax positions. This observation can be explained by the mechanoreceptor and nociceptor reflex mechanisms (WYKE, 1979b).

Disturbances in the acromioclavicular joints can induce reflexogenic tendomyoses in the anterior serratus muscle, the trapezius muscle, the biceps brachii muscle, the coracobrachialis muscle, and the hand and finger extensors (Brügger, 1977).

The sternal syndrome may not only lead to tendomyoses of the musculature of the shoulder, neck, chest wall, or arm acroparesthesias, but also to trophic disturbances of the skin. According to an important observation by Brügger (1977), it is possible that primarily brachial syndromes (including carpal tunnel syndrome and overload injuries) induce a secondary reflexogenic sternal syndrome (GERSTENBRAND et al., 1979).

3.2.3.2. Syndrome of the Trunk

Functional disturbances of the locomotive apparatus in the region of the trunk and diseases of inner organs can lead to arthrotendomyotic syn-

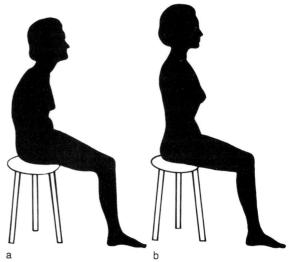

a   b

Fig. **42**. (a) Slouched position, (b) erect (straight) thorax position (after *Brügger*, 1977).

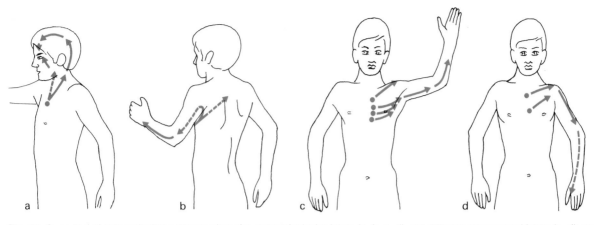

Fig. **43**. Overview of pain radiation patterns when the sternoclavicular joints (**a, b, c, d**) and different sternocostal joints (**c, d**) are irritated through puncture (*Brügger*).

dromes via nociceptive and somatomotoric reflexes (Brügger, 1965).

A thorough knowledge of soft tissue anatomy, palpatory determination of painful tendomyoses, analysis of body posture and movement patterns, and local infiltration with anesthetics in the originally disturbed joints (apophyseal joints, costovertebral joints) all help to distinguish the primarily functional disturbances of the locomotive apparatus from the primarily organic diseases (WYKE, 1979a).

It is known that a primary segmental dysfunction of the locomotive apparatus can cause referred pain in the inner organs (SCHWARZ, 1974b). The reverse is also observed, that is, diseases of inner organs can reflexogenically induce tendomyotic changes (somatovisceral, viscerosomatic reflexes [Korr, 1975]).

3.2.2.3. Syndromes of the Lower Body

According to Brügger, the functional unit of the lower body consists of the thoracolumbar spine with its posterior and anterior back and abdominal muscles, the pelvis, and the legs.

Abnormal mechanical strains on the locomotive apparatus in the lumbosacral junction evoke tendomyotic reactions in the abdominal, pelvic, and leg muscles. Brügger believes that this can result in edematous swelling and reactive inflammatory changes in the regions of the tendinous insertions, tendinous sheaths, and interstitial tissue of the musculature (FASSBENDER and WEGNER, 1973; FASSBENDER, 1980). The efficiency of the locomotive apparatus is further decreased by the nociceptive somatomotoric inhibiting effect. Brügger explains with this mechanism the numerous lumbar algesias and leg pains and partially explains the syndromes of the small pelvis (iliopsoas muscle).

Subcutaneous inflammatory processes, hemorrhages, and scars can also cause arthrotendomyotic signs (REYNOLDS, 1981).

The differentiation between cause and effect is difficult until the reflexogenic arthrotendomyotic manifestations are recognized as such and can be differentiated from the real focus of disease.

Stimulation of the apophyseal joints in the thoracolumbar and the lumbosacral junctions can cause pain in the abdominal wall muscles and the paravertebral and leg muscles according to their tendomyotic pattern (Fig. **44**).

Radiation of pain into the abdominal organs is also described (SCHWARZ, 1974b).

3.2.3.4. Symphyseal Syndrome

It is observed that the infiltration of the symphysis with local anesthetics can lead to the immediate disappearance of pain in the small pelvis or legs. This would indicate that both the symphysis and the pelvis can play a role in disease. With irritation of the symphysis or with functional disturbances of the pelvis, tendomyotic reactions are observed in the paravertebral muscles (symphyseal lumbar algesias), the muscles of the pelvis and the abdomen (symphyseal abdominal wall pain), and leg muscles (quadriceps femoris muscle, sartorius muscle, tensor fasciae latae muscle) (Brügger, 1962, 1977) (Fig. **45**).

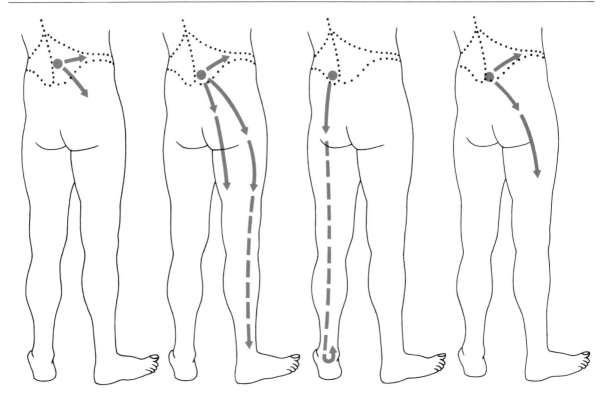

Fig. **44**. Pain radiation patterns when puncturing different apophyseal joints (after *Brügger*, 1962).

It is often impossible to distinguish the primary symphyseal disturbance from secondary, reflexogenically affected, painful changes of the ligaments and tendoperiosteal tissue of the symphysis, that is, caused by disturbances in the thoracic spine.

In the slouched posture, as described by Brügger (Fig. **46**), the balance of the synergism between the sacrospinalis muscle and the abdominal wall muscles is displaced in favor of the abdominal muscles, which in turn can lead to irritation of the symphysis. In order to recognize a true radicular syndrome, it is necessary to understand the reflexogenic tendomyotic reactions resulting from irritation of the symphysis or a slouched position (Fig. **47**).

The longissimus thoracis muscle between the sacrum and the central thoracic spine is hypotonically tendomyotic (pain between the shoulder blades and in the lumbar region). To prevent backward tilt, the iliopsoas muscle contracts. The tensor fasciae latae muscle, the sartorius muscle, and the rectus femoris muscle act synergistically. The ischiocrural calf muscles and peroneal muscles become rather painfully hypotonic.

When a tendomyotic pain syndrome develops in this fashion, it can very well simulate a radicular lumbar sciatica.

The palpatory examination of the affected muscle groups is to be performed in the slouched, erect, or supine positions. The tendomyotic reactions often disappear with upright posture.

Figure **48** gives an overview of the nonradicular pattern of pain radiation when different joint capsules are irritated.

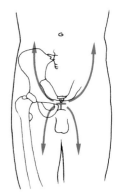

Fig. **45**. Pain radiation with irritation of the symphysis (after *Brügger*).

3.2.4. Tender Points

Osteopathic physicians postulate that the "somatic joint dysfunction" is the basis of the segmental diagnosis and therapy (JONES, 1981; KORR, 1975; MITCHELL et al., 1979). This term is defined as the impaired or altered physiological function of related components within the somatic (body framework) system: the skeletal, arthrodial, and myofascial structures, and the related vascular, lymphatic, and neural elements. As a result of this definition, the "osteopathic lesion" was registered with the International Classification of Diseases under the number 739.

The tender points (JONES, 1964; KELLGREN, 1938) provide important information for the diagnosis of joint function, both of the apophyseal and peripheral joints and consequently the reflexogenic changes in soft tissue.

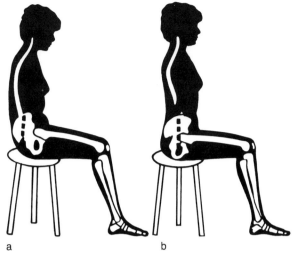

Fig. 46. A torque acting in the posterior direction when the patient is in the slouched position (**a**). The disappearance of the torque in the pelvic region when patient is sitting erect (**b**) (after *Brügger*).

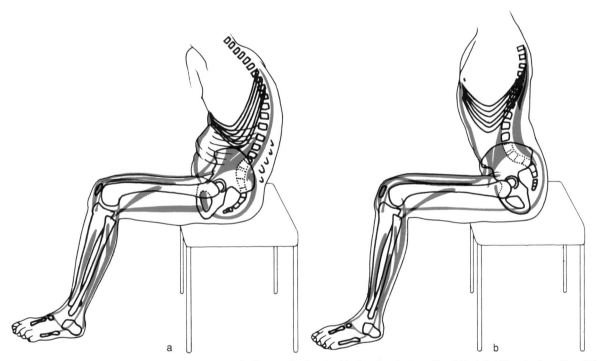

Fig. **47**. Muscles involved in extension of the trunk (red), muscles involved in the slouched position (blue). (**a**) Slouched position, (**b**) erect position (after *Brügger*).

The tender points which are painful upon pressure (stabbing pain), are usually found in the proximity of the affected joint as swollen, flat regions in specific parts of the body. They are located in the deeper muscle layers, and their size does not normally exceed 1 cm in diameter.

With spondylogenic dysfunction, they often appear multiply, primarily in the paravertebral region (articular processes), but also on the anterior side of the trunk (Fig. **49**).

Tender points have been described for all joint dysfunctions. Even with subclinical disturbances,

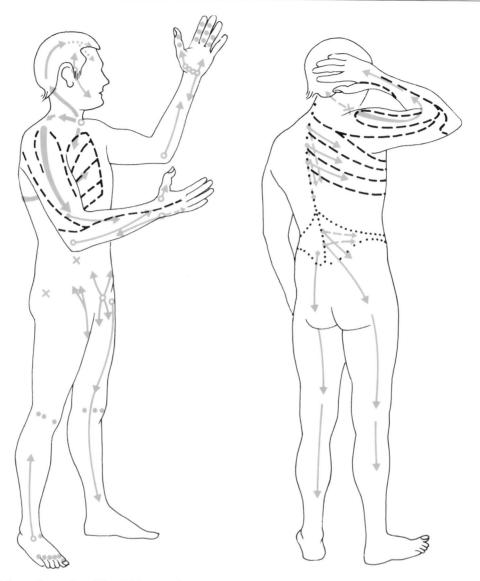

Fig. **48**. Pain radiation patterns when different joint capsules are irritated by way of puncture (after *Brügger*, 1962).

they can be demonstrated by the careful palpation (compare latent phase of the intervertebral insufficiency according to SCHMORL and JUNGHANNS [1968]). The results of the positional examination indicate the direction of the manual therapeutic approach. When the joint is positioned so that pain is absent, the painfulness of the related tender point decreases significantly, and sometimes diminished tissue tension can be noted with palpation. After proper therapy, they are no longer evident (compare the definition of the zone of irritation).

The understanding of the segmental diagnosis and the experience with soft tissue palpation led to the

"muscle energy" (MITCHELL et al., 1979) and later the "strain and counterstrain" techniques (JONES, 1964, 1981). These two methods are similar to the muscle facilitation and inhibition techniques (LEWIT, 1981).

3.2.5. Spondylogenic Reflex Syndrome

Empirical clinical observations showed that relationships exist between the axial skeleton and the peripheral soft tissues which are not easily explained on the basis of radicular, vascular, or humoral reasoning. SUTTER (1975) defines these clinical, empirically determined interrelationships as the spondylogenic reflex syndromes (SRS).

Being mediated through the reflexogenic pathway of the CNS, the SRS is defined as the reproducible, causative relationship between the reciprocal functionally abnormal position (segmental dysfunction) of skeletal parts of the axial skeleton and the local, anatomically determined noninflammatory rheumatic soft tissue changes. The term "functionally abnormal position" (segmental dysfunction) is understood as a disturbance of the so-called inner function of the vertebral unit. The well-balanced interaction between the bony structures (skull, vertebrae, pelvis) and the corresponding muscletendon apparatus is impaired. MAIGNE (1970) describes these disturbances as "dérangements intervertebrales mineurs."

The functionally abnormal position (segmental dysfunction), however, is not always identical to those changes of the skeletal parts that can be detected spatially on radiographs (such as scoliosis and deformities,). The dysfunction leads to reversible, objectively demonstrable impairments of mobility in the appropriate skeletal segment.

The afferent source of the SRS is primarily the intervertebral joints. Reflexogenically induced disturbances (via CNS) in the appropriate peripheral soft tissue can develop (WALLER, 1975) as a result of permanently suprathreshold stimulations of the numerous mechano- and nociceptive receptors in the joint capsules and ligamentous structures (WYKE, 1976b).

The first demonstrable clinical manifestation is the so-called zone of irritation (CAVIEZEL, 1976), also known as segmental point (SELL, 1969), paravertebral point (MAIGNE, 1970), or TP (JONES, 1981).

These are painful swellings, tender upon pressure, and detectable with palpation, located in the musculofascial tissue in topographically well-defined sites (refer to chapter 6). The average size varies from 0.5 to 1 cm, and the main characteristic is the absolutely timed and qualitative linkage to the extent of the functionally abnormal position (segmental dysfunction). As long as a disturbance exists, the zones of irritation can be identified, yet disappear immediately after the removal of the disturbance. This is extremely important for therapeutic control. It is emphasized that one deals with a clinical-palpatory term. To date, no anatomic-histological substantiation for the zones of irritation has been found.

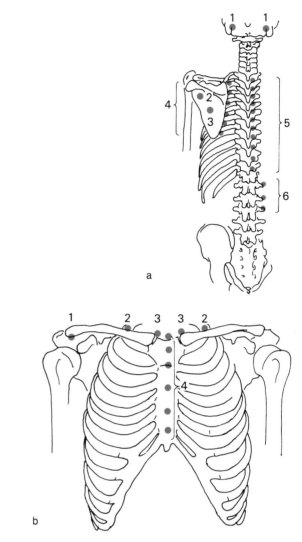

Fig. **49. a**) Localization of tender points, posteriorly (examples) (after *Jones*, 1981). 1: C_1; 2: T_2; 3: T_3; 4: ribs; 5: T_1-T_{12}; 6: L_1-L_3.
b) Localization of the tender points, anteriorly (examples) (after *Jones*, 1981). 1: Acromioclavicular joint; 2: C_7; 3: sternoclavicular joint; 4: T_1-T_6.

Among the most important causes of the functionally abnormal position (segmental dysfunction) are uncoordinated movement, trauma, muscular imbalance, acute and chronic mechanical overload of the vertebrae, and osteo-ligamentous insufficiency. Additionally, one must consider inflammatory, arthrotic-degenerative irritations as well as neoplastic infiltrations to be pathological afferences from the intervertebral joints (NORTHUP, 1966).

The functionally abnormal position (segmental dysfunction) in a vertebral unit results in the reflexogenic pathological change of the soft tissue, the most important being the "myotendinoses," which can be identified by palpation.

3.2.5.1. Myotendinoses

The healthy muscle displays normal plasticity and homogeneity and the individual muscle bundles cannot be differentiated from each other by palpation.

Myotendinotic changes are characterized by increased permanent tone, elevated consistency, resistance and decreased plasticity. A whole muscle or only a few muscle bundles in the longitudinal direction can be affected. When palpating perpendicularly to the muscle fibers with average pressure myoses or myotendinoses are painful and can easily be differentiated from the surrounding area of the same muscle not immediately affected. Myotendinotic changes can be palpated from the origin to the insertion of the muscle. "Nervous misinformation" of certain muscle bundles (FASSBENDER, 1980) arriving in the reflexogenic pathway is responsible for the origin of the involuntary isometric increase of tonus in the muscle bundle (Fig. **50**).

It is possible, but not proven, that these tendomyotic changes of a muscle are simply the result of or are caused by segmental dysfunction, which would partially explain the so-called noninflammatory soft tissue rheumatism (Fig. **51**).

Myosis is the state of increased painful changes in texture that can be caused by pressure or that can appear spontaneously. Myoses exist mostly in the center of the muscle mass. Often they are found at

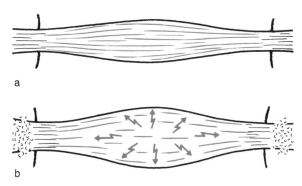

a

b

Fig. 51. **a**) normal muscle, **b**) tendomyotically altered muscle (schematic).

sites where the course of the whole muscle is changed or at the free muscle borders (that is, trapezius muscle, pectoralis major muscle).

With continued, nonphysiological stimulatory impulses and the presence of permanently increased tonus, degenerative changes appear (FASSBENDER, 1973, 1980), resulting in the damage of the muscle fibers (Fig. **52**).

Attachment-tendinoses are local swellings of tendons that are well defined at the origin and insertion and are extremely painful upon palpatory pressure in the direction of the inserting tendinous fibers. The typical hallmark is their mirror image appearance. In addition to these typical sites at the points of origin and insertion, tendinoses can also appear at the muscle and tendon junction.

Abnormal growth of the mesenchymal cells (FASSBENDER, 1980; FASSBENDER and WEGNER, 1973) caused by relative hypoxia can be detected morphologically (Fig. **52**).

Due to their reflexogenic nature, the appearance of tendinoses and myoses is delayed. They disappear following a latent period (thus called "latent zones" by SUTTER) once the causative disturbance has been eliminated. This is an important differential diagnostic quality distinguishing them from the zones of irritation. Clinically, they must be differentiated from those myotendinoses caused by other mechanisms (such as trauma).

A certain muscle contains the same amount of defined longitudinal sections that can independently undergo tendomyotic changes in a set sequence. Such a clinical muscle unit with the corresponding tendons is named a myotenone. Slender muscles represent a single myotenone. Broad, flat, and fan-shaped muscles comprise several myotenones (Fig. **53**).

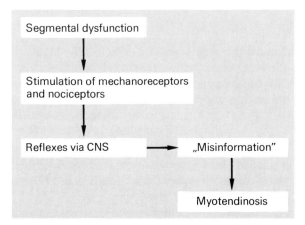

Fig. **50**. Development of myotendinosis (after *Fassbender*, 1980).

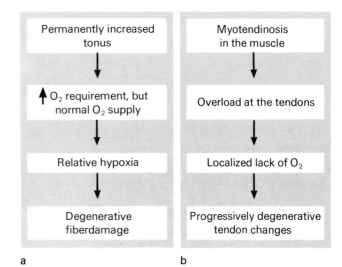

Permanently increased tonus	Myotendinosis in the muscle
↓	↓
↑ O_2 requirement, but normal O_2 supply	Overload at the tendons
↓	↓
Relative hypoxia	Localized lack of O_2
↓	↓
Degenerative fiberdamage	Progressively degenerative tendon changes

Fig. 52. Pathogenesis of the noninflammatory soft tissue rheumatism (after *Fassbender*): **a**) in muscle-myosis, **b**) in tendinous portions (tendinosis).

a   b

Clinical experience shows that certain axial skeletal parts are correlated with certain myotenones, which can be reproduced symmetrically, qualitatively, and objectively. A functional disturbance in one vertebral unit initiates myotendinosis simultaneously in the empirically correlated myotenones. Since the spondylogenic-reflexogenic myotendinoses can be routinely located, they are collectively termed "systematic myotendinosis" (SUTTER and FRÖHLICH, 1981; TRAVELL and RINZLER, 1952). The primary functionally abnormal position of a vertebral unit, followed by myotendinotic changes represents the primary SRS.

Under certain circumstances additional secondary, tertiary, and other SRSs can develop in a chain reaction. Thus, factors such as the basic composition of the spine, type of carriage, motion, and muscle, muscular imbalance, muscle strength, and joint function play an important role. In clinical practice we most often find an inherently complex picture. Often, it is not possible to determine the causative primary SRS, especially in patients with chronic conditions; it may have healed already. In those cases the induced secondary and other SRSs are considered primary (TRAVELL, 1981).

In order to establish the correct diagnosis and to initiate the appropriate therapy, careful examination techniques and precise anatomical knowledge are necessary.

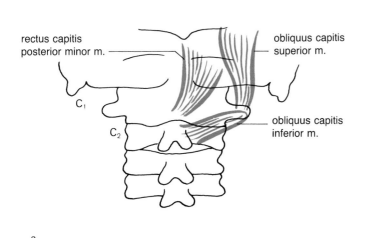

rectus capitis posterior minor m.

obliquus capitis superior m.

C_1

C_2

obliquus capitis inferior m.

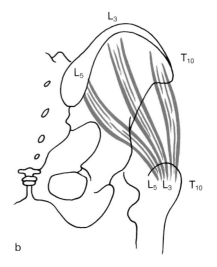

L_3

L_5

T_{10}

L_5 L_3 T_{10}

a   b

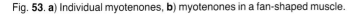

Fig. 53. **a**) Individual myotenones, **b**) myotenones in a fan-shaped muscle.

4. The Clinical Correlation of the Reflexes Associated with the Nociceptors and Mechanoreceptors – the Spondylogenic Reflex Syndrome

The clinical symptoms of pain, be it spontaneous pain or pain due to palpatory pressure, are defined by SUTTER (1974, 1975) as the SRS (see chapter 3).

The authors were likewise able to observe the so-called systematic myotendinoses with a functionally abnormal position or segmental dysfunction involving the individual apophyseal, occipital-atlanto-axial, and sacroiliac joints. During the course of therapeutic intervention, improvement of these systematic myotendinoses could be seen in the individual patient. One therefore assumed that, in addition to other helpful physical and therapeutic procedures, the mechanical correction of the vertebral unit plays the primary role (SCHMORL and JUNGHANNS, 1968).

The results of articular neurology, according to WYKE, present new views contributing significantly to the diagnostic and therapeutic understanding of manual medicine.

The authors found in a clinical study of adolescents that the absence of pain is not identical with absence of soft tissue findings. It is well known that systematic myotendinoses can often be detected with palpation in those individuals subjectively free of complaints. According to our understanding, this situation is to be considered pathological and correlates with the latent state of intervertebral insufficiency (SCHMORL and JUNGHANNS, 1968). Using the experimental work by WYKE for comparison, one would equate this with the tonic reflexogenic influence of the type I mechanoreceptors upon the motoneurons of the axial musculature and musculature of the extremities. The fact that pain-inducing nociceptors demonstrate a significantly higher threshold than pain-inhibiting mechanoreceptors explains the time delay for the subjective perception of the emotional disturbance presenting the patient with pain. In this situation as well, however, the nociceptive stimulatory conduction can be inhibited presynaptically by adequate stimuli of the mechanoreceptors (mainly type II).

It is very likely that this neurophysiological mechanism plays as important a role in the manual therapeutic treatment as the mechanical correction of the segmental dysfunction. Figures **54** and **55** attempt to present this model schematically.

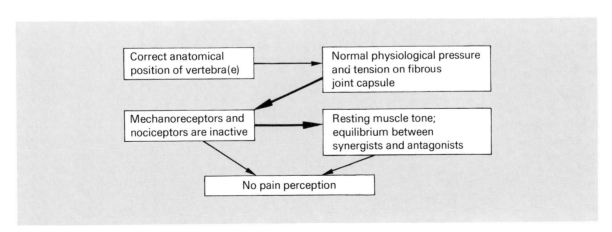

Fig. **54**. Model for the receptor activity when vertebrae are in the correct position.

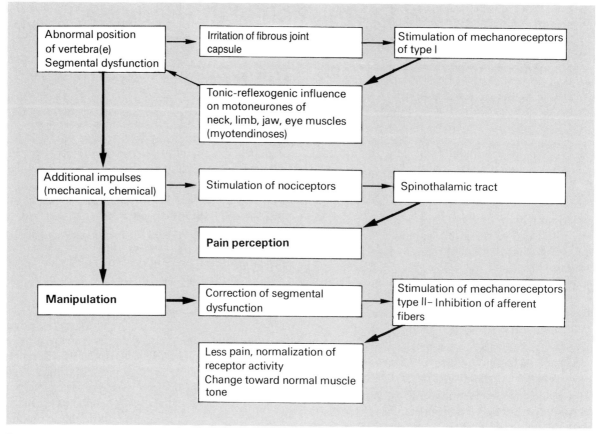

Fig. **55**. Model for receptor activity when vertebrae are in abnormal position (segmental dysfunction).

5. General Principles of Palpation

A thorough, well-founded knowledge of anatomy is necessary in order to understand the nature and principles of the SRS and to be able to apply it to the patient (see chapter 3). From a manual medicine viewpoint, the anatomy requires a three-dimensional understanding that, depending on the individual anatomical situation, can be perceived by palpation. The anatomical structure being examined should be palpated from its origin to its insertion. It should be a known fact that healthy structures often cannot be distinguished from each other. A pathologically altered structure (myotendinosis, ligamentosis), however, can be exactly differentiated from the surrounding healthy tissue. Palpation is started at that site where the patient localizes the pain, be it spontaneous pain or pain upon pressure. Normally, the patient finds the pain to be restricted to a specific point, area, or even a whole tract. Pain can be present in the resting or contracted muscle. It is our task to identify the painful structure. The three-dimensional anatomical perception is of utmost importance in the examination. When following a structure, one stays at the same palpatory level. The homologous origin and insertion tendinoses must be present. The identification takes place by exclusion, whereby one must always picture which muscles, ligaments and other structures are located above and next to each other in that specific topographical region.

Principles of Palpation:

Palpation can be viewed as objective, examiner's sensation; or subjective, patient's sensation. Objective palpation, guided by sound anatomical knowledge, applies adequate pressure with regard to area, force, and direction.

Requirements for an Adequate Palpation:

- The painful sites indicated by the patient must be localized and palpated precisely.

- The pressure used for palpation must be large enough for the palpating finger to feel the hard, bony structures.

- The palpating force must act along the tendon to reach the place of insertion at the bone. This technical detail is of crucial importance for a satisfactory palpatory result.

- Comparison of symmetrical skeletal structures is not to be applied, since the disturbance is always qualitatively symmetrical and often quantitatively symmetrical or very nearly so. Thus, comparison must be limited to the same side, that is, to locations with the same anatomical arrangement and sites undergoing no changes.

- In order to prevent confusion, similar changes of adjacent structures must be differentiated. This is achieved by palpating the course, shape, and the opposite poles of the attachments (origin-insertion) of these structures.

- Myotendinotic changes in the muscle are identified by using a pressing and stroking type of palpation, which is performed perpendicular to the direction of the fibers and is thus compared with a so-called ploughing type of palpation. Consequently, this examination is repeated until reaching the origins and insertions.

Before the student gets confused with too many details of the SRS symptomatology, we would like to emphasize once more that the palpation should be practiced and carried out as precisely as possible. Unfortunately, we ourselves have experienced that many a negative palpatory finding was due to improper palpatory technique and insufficient anatomical knowledge.

6. Zones of Irritation

The nature of the zone of irritation has been discussed in chapter 3. Since the functionally abnormal position, segmental dysfunction, of a skeletal part cannot be visualized as such, it must be diagnosed by using its clinical presentation as well as its improvement after spontaneous or manual and therapeutic correction of the basic disturbance.

Therefore the zone of irritation acquires an important, as yet unmentioned property. Being an indicator for the spatially and functionally abnormal position of an axial skeletal part, the zone of irritation reacts by either increased or decreased intensity when the abnormal position is altered by specifically changing the relationship of the actual skeletal parts to each other. This process is also an important differential diagnostic technique for the latent zone (compare chapter 3) that can be provoked and thus is called the test of provocation. The actual procedure is not the same for all zones of irritation and for didactic reasons, is described

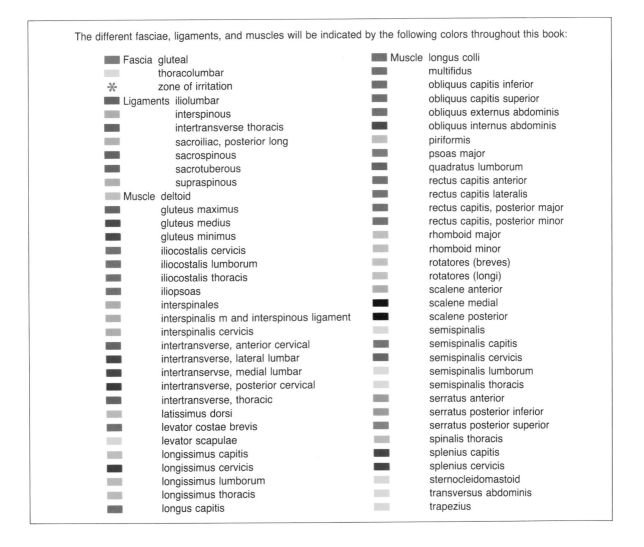

The different fasciae, ligaments, and muscles will be indicated by the following colors throughout this book:

Fascia gluteal
    thoracolumbar
    zone of irritation
Ligaments iliolumbar
    interspinous
    intertransverse thoracis
    sacroiliac, posterior long
    sacrospinous
    sacrotuberous
    supraspinous
Muscle deltoid
    gluteus maximus
    gluteus medius
    gluteus minimus
    iliocostalis cervicis
    iliocostalis lumborum
    iliocostalis thoracis
    iliopsoas
    interspinales
    interspinalis m and interspinous ligament
    interspinalis cervicis
    intertransverse, anterior cervical
    intertransverse, lateral lumbar
    intertransevse, medial lumbar
    intertransverse, posterior cervical
    intertransverse, thoracic
    latissimus dorsi
    levator costae brevis
    levator scapulae
    longissimus capitis
    longissimus cervicis
    longissimus lumborum
    longissimus thoracis
    longus capitis

Muscle longus colli
    multifidus
    obliquus capitis inferior
    obliquus capitis superior
    obliquus externus abdominis
    obliquus internus abdominis
    piriformis
    psoas major
    quadratus lumborum
    rectus capitis anterior
    rectus capitis lateralis
    rectus capitis, posterior major
    rectus capitis, posterior minor
    rhomboid major
    rhomboid minor
    rotatores (breves)
    rotatores (longi)
    scalene anterior
    scalene medial
    scalene posterior
    semispinalis
    semispinalis capitis
    semispinalis cervicis
    semispinalis lumborum
    semispinalis thoracis
    serratus anterior
    serratus posterior inferior
    serratus posterior superior
    spinalis thoracis
    splenius capitis
    splenius cervicis
    sternocleidomastoid
    transversus abdominis
    trapezius

along with the palpatory technique of the individual zones of irritation.

In addition to the differential diagnostic significance, knowledge of the zone of irritation and of its reaction upon provocational testing is of decisive therapeutic consequence. With a well-planned manipulative strategy, the vertebrae in question are acted upon in such a direction as to achieve the decrease of the zone of irritation.

6.1.   Zones of Irritation in the Cervical Spine Region

C_0–C_1

These two zones of irritation, situated in the occipital region, are related to the positional arrangement of the occiput and the atlas (Figs. **56, 57, 58**). They are located as follows.

C_0 is lateral and superior to, and C_1 is medial and inferior to the superior end of the mastoid notch (the bony part without muscles between the splenius capitis muscle and the obliquus capitis superior muscle).

When the atlanto-occipital joint is in an abnormal position, these two zones of irritation are always present. Differentiation from other surrounding tendinoses is only possible with the help of provocative examination (see later).

The C_1-zone of irritation can also be palpated at the lateral aspect of the transverse process of the atlas. The differentiation, however, from tendinoses of the numerous other muscles originating at this location is very difficult.

C_2–C_6

The zone of irritation located at the superior articular process is of practical importance. Since the muscular insertions at the transverse processes are often painful, the irritation zones in that region are only of theoretical significance.

For palpation, four fingers of the hand are placed over the spinous processes of C_2–C_6 and then reach in a hooklike manner for the strong semispinalis capitis muscle. One perceives a groove formed by the semispinalis capitis muscle and the longissimus capitis muscle. The fingers should be in as close a contact with the bony structures as possible and should be able to feel the slight protuberanu of the superior articular process. In the neutral position, the superior articular process of C_2 is one finger width below the occiput and about one finger width superior to the inferior edge of the spinous process of C_2. The superior articular processes of C_3 and C_4 are each one finger width below. With maximal extension of the head, the zone of irritation of C_4 is located at the lowest point of the concave cervical spine, whereas that of C_5 is one and a half finger widths below that of C_4 and two finger widths superior to the spinous process. The zone of irritation of C_6 is one finger width below that of C_5.

Since the head of the seated and totally relaxed patient can be moved in any direction with the nonpalpating hand (examiner is positioned behind the patient), fine joint play of the intervertebral joints can easily be examined with the finger, further facilitating orientation.

C_7

The zone of irritation is more difficult to palpate, mainly due to the strong fibers of the trapezius muscle (descending portion) and the long, strong back muscles.

The transverse and the spinous processes of C_7 (vertebra prominens) are located first. The zone of irritation is situated two finger widths above the spinous process and about one finger width medial to the tip of the transverse process.

Provocative testing: All zones of irritation in the cervical spine region react upon provocative testing. A decrease of pain perception or any tissue change indicates the appropriate therapeutic direction for the segment being examined. It is to be noticed, that most of the abnormal positions in the cervical region take place in the posterior direction. For instance, the zone of irritation increases posteriorly upon provocative testing and decreases anteriorly.

Procedure: The index or middle finger rests over the zone of irritation applying constant pressure. The pressure is such that the patient can barely feel the pain. The other hand embraces the parietal region of the head and conducts all possible physiological motions significant for this segment.

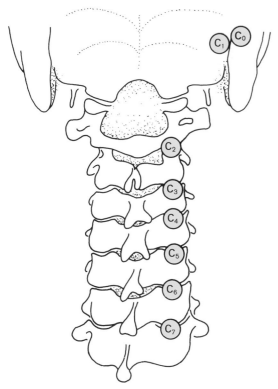

Fig. 56. Zones of irritation in the cervical spine region.

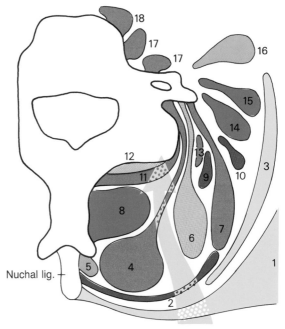

Fig. 57. Cross-section of the central cervical spine. The arrow indicates the access to the zone of irritation (after *Sutter*).

1: Trapezius m	10: Splenius cervicis m
2: Splenius capitis m	11: Multifidus m
3: Sternocleidomastoid m	12: Rotatores muscles
4: Semispinalis capitis m	13: Iliocostalis cervicis m
5: Interspinalis cervicis m	14: Scalene posterior m
6: Longissimus capitis m	15: Scalene medius m
7: Levator scapulae m	16: Scalene anterior m
8: Semispinalis cervicis m	17: Longus capitis m
9: Longissimus cervicis m	18: Longus colli m

1: Longus colli m (inferior portion)
2: Anterior cervical intertransverse m
3: Scalene anterior m
4: Posterior cervical intertransverse m
   (lateral portion)
5: Scalene medius m
   Levator scapulae m
   Splenius cervicis m
   Iliocostalis cervicis m
   Longissimus cervicis and capitis m
6: Posterior cervical intertransverse m
   (medial portion)
7: Longissimus capitis m
8: Semispinalis capitis m
9: Rotatores muscles
10: Multifidus m
11: Semispinalis cervicis m
12: Interspinalis cervicis m

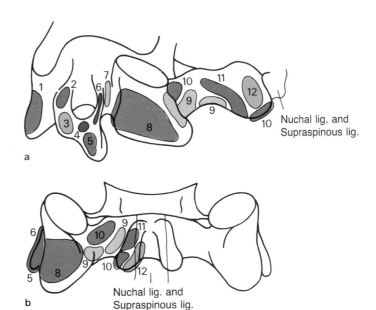

Fig. 58. Schematic representation of the muscle origins and insertions at the mid-cervical vertebra.

6.2.   Zones of Irritation in the Region of the Thoracic Spine, Ribs, and Sternum

The relaxed patient is in the prone position. For better control, the thoracic kyphosis is accentuated by adjusting the examination table. The patient's arms hang either freely over the edge of the table or the elbows are spread so that the shoulder blades draw somewhat apart from the midline.

Thoracic Spine

In the thoracic spine, the irritational zone at the transverse process is of practical importance (Fig. **59**). It can be located as follows: the thumb moves laterally along the rib toward the transverse process of the thoracic vertebra. Two to three finger widths lateral to the spinous process it meets the massive muscle structure of the longissimus system, which is gently pushed medially. During this procedure, the thumb reaches a region where the rib disappears below the transverse process (Fig. **40**). The zone of irritation (1 to 2 cm long) located here presents itself as a nonmoveable, painful threshold. One should note that the palpatory pressure is applied in the lateral direction in order to avoid confusion with tendinoses of the longissimus thoracis muscle.

To determine the correct level, we orient ourselves at the spinous processes. In the central thoracic spine region, the distance between the inferior margin of the spinous process and the superior margin of the transverse process of the same vertebra measures three finger widths and decreases to two finger widths when moving either superiorly or inferiorly (verify on a skeleton).

Provocative testing: The palpating thumb remains at the zone of irritation, while the hypothenar of the other hand presses on the spinous process from the opposite side. If the zone of irritation does not decrease, pressure from either a superior or inferior direction is applied. Consequently, the behavior of the zone of irritation allows differentiation between an abnormal rotatory position and a possible ventralization of the vertebra.

Ribs

The zones of irritation at the ribs lie in the region of the costal angle between the longissimus thoracis muscle and the iliocostalis thoracis muscle (Fig. **59**).

The position of the patient for this examination is the same as for that of the thoracic spine.

About two finger widths lateral to the transverse process, the thumb presses vertically trying to get between both muscles to establish as close a contact with the bony structures as possible; the direction is posteroinferior. If a zone of irritation is present, little pressure is sufficient to cause pain.

Provocative testing: The thumb rests at the zone of irritation, exerting constant minimal pressure sufficient to cause pain. The index finger of the other hand is placed with its whole surface over the corresponding rib, with the palpatory pressure in the sternal direction. If the zone of irritation does not decrease, pressure is changed toward the transverse process.

Sternum

When examining the zones of irritation of the ribs, the sternal zones of irritation should also be inspected. They are situated on the midline between the jugular notch and the xiphoid process (Fig. **60**). Objective palpatory perception is often impossible, and thus one relies on the patient's specification about pain.

These zones of irritation also react upon provocative testing. The procedure is similar to that performed for the ribs.

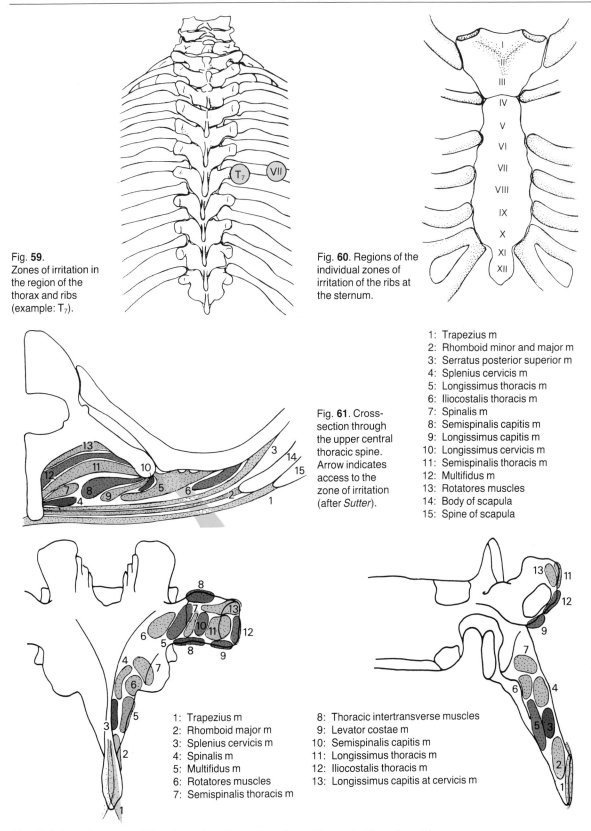

Fig. **59**. Zones of irritation in the region of the thorax and ribs (example: T_7).

Fig. **60**. Regions of the individual zones of irritation of the ribs at the sternum.

Fig. **61**. Cross-section through the upper central thoracic spine. Arrow indicates access to the zone of irritation (after *Sutter*).

1: Trapezius m
2: Rhomboid minor and major m
3: Serratus posterior superior m
4: Splenius cervicis m
5: Longissimus thoracis m
6: Iliocostalis thoracis m
7: Spinalis m
8: Semispinalis capitis m
9: Longissimus capitis m
10: Longissimus cervicis m
11: Semispinalis thoracis m
12: Multifidus m
13: Rotatores muscles
14: Body of scapula
15: Spine of scapula

1: Trapezius m
2: Rhomboid major m
3: Splenius cervicis m
4: Spinalis m
5: Multifidus m
6: Rotatores muscles
7: Semispinalis thoracis m

8: Thoracic intertransverse muscles
9: Levator costae m
10: Semispinalis capitis m
11: Longissimus thoracis m
12: Iliocostalis thoracis m
13: Longissimus capitis at cervicis m

Fig. **62**. Schematic representation of muscle origin and insertions at the central thoracic vertebra.

6.3. Zones of Irritation in the Lumbar Spine Region

L_1-L_4

In the L_1-L_4 region, the zones of irritation located at the costal processes are of practical significance.

The relaxed patient rests in the prone position on the examination table. The palpating finger reaches and follows the iliocostalis muscle laterally, including the whole sacrospinal system, and continues between this muscle and the inferior abdominal muscles, finally terminating at the tip of the transverse process. If the patient is not obese, good contact with the bone is possible, and one searches for pathological painful resistance. With muscular or obese patients, one relies rather on provocative testing and the consequent manifestation and alteration of pain (Fig. **64**).

The transverse process of L_4 is normally located at the level of the iliac crest. The transverse processes of L_3, L_2, and L_1 lie each two finger widths superior to the vertebra below, respectively. In other words, they can be found at the level of the lower pole of the spinous process of the vertebra immediately above. Due to its anatomical position, the costal process of L_5 cannot be palpated easily (Fig. **63**).

It is often impossible to make a distinction between the numerous tendinoses of the lateral lumbar intertransverse muscles and the quadratus lumborum muscle. Thus, one should look either for spondylogenically correlated tendinoses, for instance in the gluteus medius and gluteus maximus muscles, or for the mirror image tendinoses at the opposing poles of the involved muscles.

The zones of irritation are localized at the lateral aspect of the inferior pole of the spinous processes. The differentiation between tendinoses of the latissimus dorsi muscle and the posterior inferior serratus muscle is only possible with provocative testing. The zones of irritation at the superior articular processes are mentioned here for completeness and are only of theoretical value due to their proximity to the mamillary processes and the corresponding origins of the transversospinal and sacrospinal musculature.

L_5

The zone of irritation of L_5 is located above the flat, posterior inferior iliac spine, which can barely be palpated. It is found one finger width lateral and inferior to the prominent posterior superior iliac spine (Fig. **63**).

Provocative testing: The thumb remains with constant pressure over the zone of irritation while the other hand rests at the thoracolumbar junction and slowly increases the pressure in an anteroinferior direction. As a result, the abnormal position of the posteriorly displaced vertebra is corrected in part; the zone of irritation decreases.

If neither pain nor palpatory manifestation decrease, one has to assume that the abnormal vertebral position is in the anterior direction. This situation is often seen as the result of the static configuration of the lumbar spine and the influence of the psoas major muscle. Diagnostically to identify this abnormal position correctly, the prone patient is positioned over a rubber ball and is asked to relax totally; the zone of irritation should decrease.

The therapeutic correction for the anteriorly displaced thoracic vertebra is achieved with the hand of an assistant, which exerts a constant pressure transabdominally on the vertebra during manipulation.

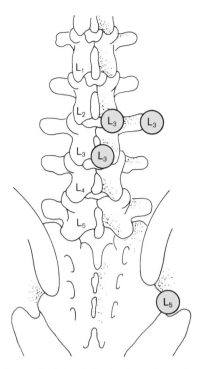

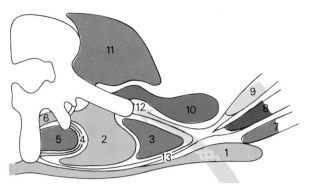

Fig. **64**. Cross-section through the lumbar spine. Arrow indicates access to the zone of irritation (after *Sutter*).

1: Latissimus dorsi m
2: Longissimus thoracis m
3: Iliocostalis lumborum m
4: Semispinalis lumborum m
5: Multifidus m
6: Rotatores muscles
7: External abdominal oblique m
8: Internal abdominal oblique m
9: Transversus abdominis m
10: Quadratus lumborum m
11: Psoas major m
12: Thoracolumbar fascia (deep layer)
13: Thoracolumbar fascia (superficial layer)

Fig. **63**. Zones of irritation in the lumbar spine region (example: L₃).

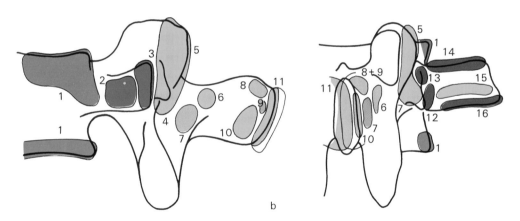

a   b

Fig. **65**. Schematic representation of muscle origins and insertions at a lumbar vertebra.

1: Psoas major m
2: Quadratus lumborum m
  (deep, anterior layer)
3: Quadratus lumborum m
  (superficial, posterior layer)
4: Longissimus lumborum m
  (medial line of insertion)
5: Longissimus thoracis m
  Semispinalis lumborum m
  Multifidus m
  Rotatores muscles (origin)
6: Rotator m (insertion)

7: Multifidus m
8: Spinalis m
9: Interspinalis lumborum m
10: Longissimus thoracis m
11: Latissimus dorsi m
12: Medial lumbar intertransverse m (origin)
13: Medial lumbar intertransverse m (insertion)
14: Lateral lumbar intertransverse m (origin)
15: Longissimus lumborum m (lateral insertions)
16: Lateral lumbar intertransverse m (insertion)

6.4.   Zones of Irritation of the Sacrum (Sacroiliac Joint) and the Pelvis

The zones of irritation of S_1–S_3 can easily be palpated by the beginner due to their anatomical location and relationship to the surrounding musculature. They react quite impressively upon provocative testing ("ventral-testing" according to SUTTER).

The zones of irritation are localized in the region of the articulating tubercle of the sacrum, between the posterior inferior iliac spine and the cornu of the sacrum. The S_1 zone of irritation lies about 1 cm medial to the posterior inferior iliac spine, the irritation zone of S_3 proximally to the sacral horn, and the irritation zone of S_2 between these two (Fig. **66**).

The relaxed patient rests in the prone position on the examination table. Before palpation is started, the bony structures, such as the iliac crest, the posterior superior iliac spine, the free lateral angle of the sacrum, and the spinous processes of L_5 and S_1 are located exactly and are marked on the skin with a pen for better orientation.

After the free lateral angle of the sacrum has been identified, the thumb that is used for palpation presses down vertically onto the amuscular bony part, right between the erector spinae and the gluteus maximus muscles. These muscles are incased in separate fasciae, almost forming a groove. This provides a close bony contact for palpation (Fig. **67a**).

Seldom are multiple zones of irritation found at the sacrum simultaneously. Since each irritational zone pattern calls for an appropriate therapeutic procedure, one must examine this region very carefully.

Provocative testing for the sacral irritational zones (sacroiliac region): The zone of irritation in the SIJ region presents itself as a distinctly doughy, painful swelling that disappears when the hypothenar of the nonpalpating hand exerts pressure on the sacrum in the anterior direction. When the hand is removed, it reappears, concomitant with stabbing pain.

During this ventralization maneuver, the thumb, that is used for palpation must remain at the irritational zone exerting constant pressure.

When examining the sacroiliac joint, the symphyseal irritational zones should be located as well (Fig. **56b**). They are situated at the junction of the symphyseal cartilage and the pubic bone. Constructing a line paramedially to the symphysis, the zone of irritation of S_1 lies at the superior pole, the zone of irritation of S_2 lies in the center, and the S_3 irritation zone lies at the inferior pole of the symphysis.

Provocative testing for the symphyseal zones of irritation: The finger rests over the zone of irritation. The ipsilaterally flexed thigh of the patient is first abducted then adducted. Since the examiner will not be able to palpate any abnormality, he has to rely on the patient's information of pain.

If the zones of irritation are confined to the sacrum only, the disturbance is very likely limited to the sacroiliac joint. However, if symphyseal irritational zones exist, a disturbance in the pelvic region is indicated (hip bones and sacrum).

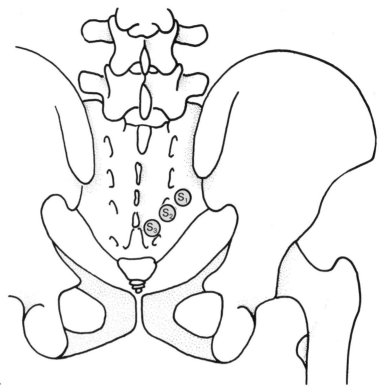

Fig. **66**. Zones of irritation at the sacrum.

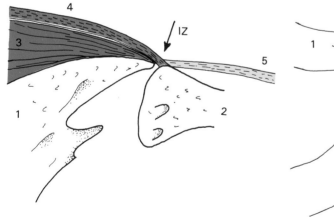

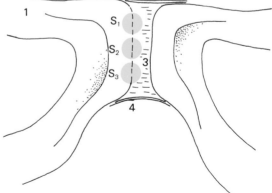

Fig. **67**. **a)** Cross-section of the sacrum and hip bones at the level of the zone of irritation S_I (ZI).

1: Hip bone
2: Sacrum
3: Gluteus maximus m.
   (superficial layer)
4: Gluteal fascia
5: Thoracolumbar fascia

Fig. **67**. **b)** Zone of irritation at the symphysis.

1: Ramus of the pubis   3: Interpubic disk
2: Superior pubic ligament   4: Arcuate ligament of the pubis

7. General Overview and List of the Different Muscles

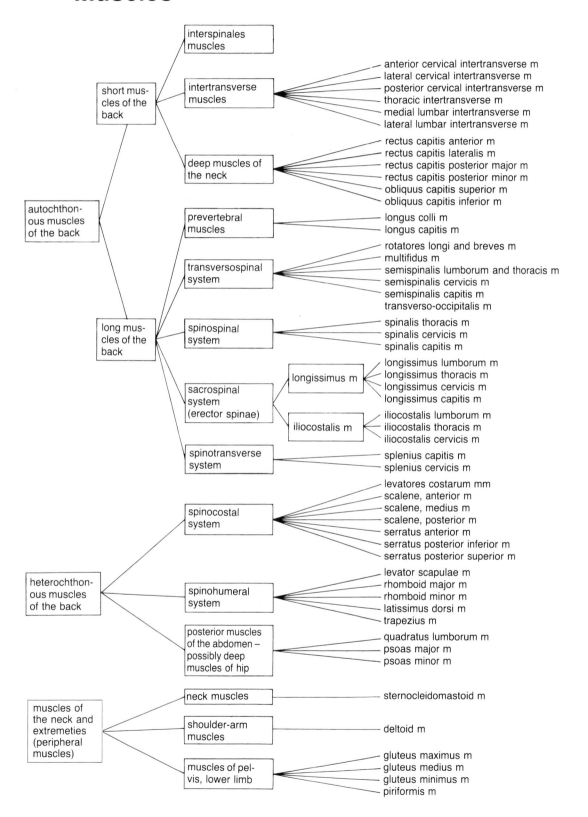

7.1.   Interspinales Muscles

These short muscles are completely present only in the cervical and lumbar spine region. In the thoracic region, these muscles exist only to T_4 and then again inferior to T_{11}. Between T_4 and T_{10}, there are normally no interspinales muscles, but there are interspinous ligaments that are, however, of the same importance for the spondylogenic event as the muscles themselves (compare the SRS correlation).

Origin: inferior surface of the spinous processes of C_2–T_3 and T_{11}–S_1.

Insertion: superior surface of the spinous process directly below the respective origin-vertebra, C_3–T_4, T_{12}–S_2.

Course and relations: practically longitudinal; in the cervical region in pairs according to the bifurcated spinous processes (Fig. **68**).

Innervation: dorsal rami of the respective spinal nerves.

Function: extension of the individual vertebrae.

Palpatory technique: In the cervical region, the muscles provide easy access when the head is slightly flexed. Generally, the origins are palpated lateroinferiorly and the insertions, laterosuperiorly.

SRS correlation: The SRS correlation of the interspinales muscles can be seen in the table to the right, but needs further explanation: it was mentioned previously that the interspinales muscles are not developed between T_3 and T_{10}. The myotenones correlated with the segments of C_0–C_6, thus corresponding to the interspinous ligaments that behave clinically and pathologically in the same manner as the muscles in the spondylogenic event.

The last column of the table lists the spondylogenic correlation of the supraspinous ligament that spreads from C_3 to S_3 above the spinous processes (Fig. **69**).

Spine	SRS Correlation			
	Interspinales muscle			Inter-spinous lig.
C_0	T_3	T_4		C_7
C_1	T_4	T_5		T_1
C_2	T_5	T_6		T_2
C_3	T_6	T_7		T_3
C_4	T_7	T_8		T_4
C_5	T_8	T_9		T_5
C_6	T_9	T_{10}		T_6
C_7	T_{10}	T_{11}		T_7
T_1	T_{11}	T_{12}		T_8
T_2	T_{12}	L_1		T_9
T_3	L_1	L_2		T_{10}
T_4	L_2	L_3		T_{11}
T_5	L_3	L_4		T_{12}
T_6	L_4	L_5		L_1
T_7	L_5	S_1		L_2
T_8	C_0	C_1		L_3
T_9	C_1	C_2		L_4
T_{10}	C_2	C_3		L_5
T_{11}	C_3	C_4		S_1
T_{12}	C_4	C_5		S_2
L_1	C_5	C_6		S_3
L_2	C_6	C_7		C_3
L_3	C_7	T_1		C_4
L_4	T_1	T_2		C_5
L_5	T_2	T_3		C_6
S_1				
S_2				
S_3				

Fig. **68**. Schematic representation of the interspinales muscles.

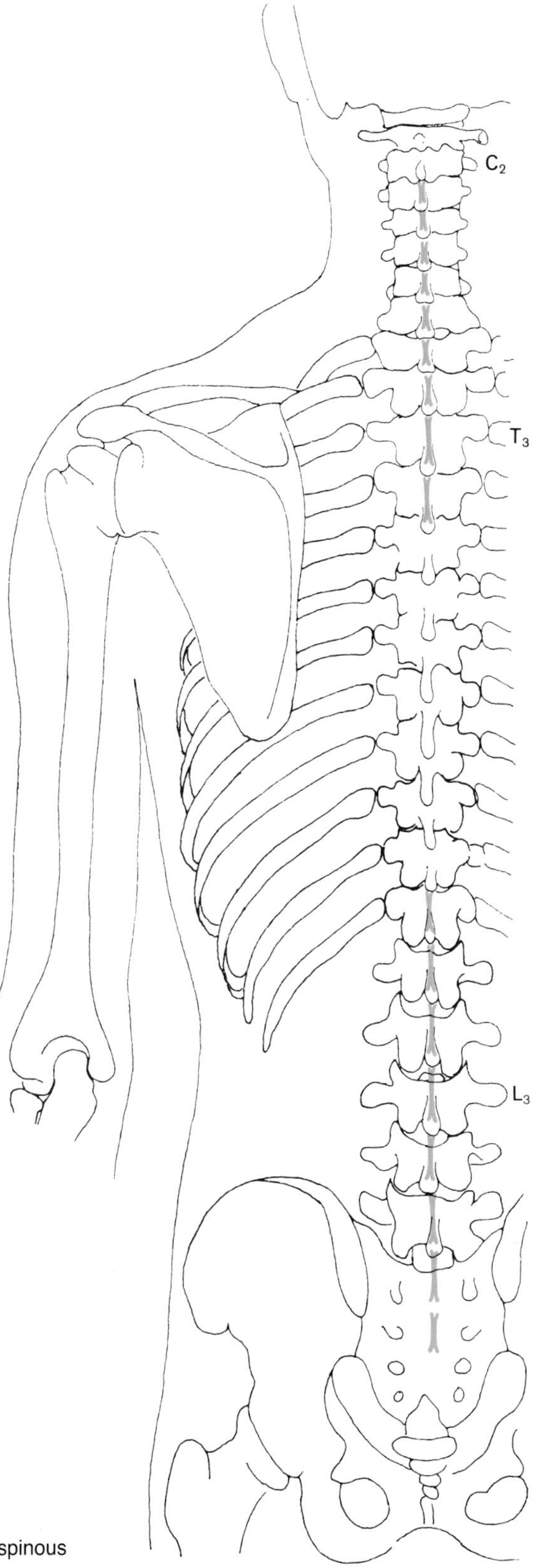

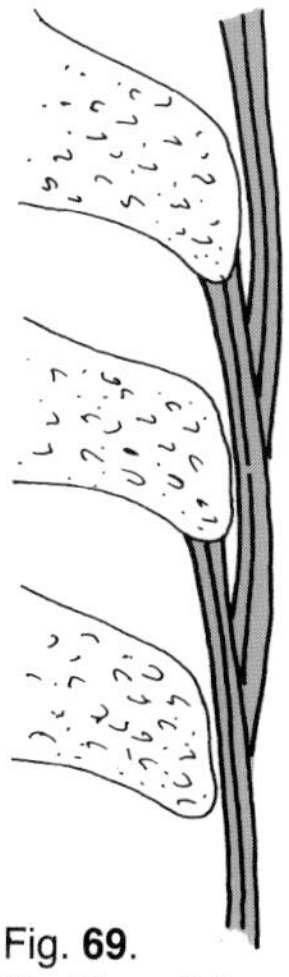

Fig. **69**.
Position of the supraspinous ligament.

7.2.   Intertransverse Muscles

Classification:

Intertransverse muscles of the cervical region: *The anterior cervical intertransverse muscles:* located anterior to the ventral ramus of the spinal nerves; together with the anterior rectus capitis muscle.

The posterior cervical intertransverse muscles (lateral part): posterior to the ventral ramus of the spinal nerves; together with the lateral rectus capitis muscle.

The posterior cervical intertransverse muscles (medial part): together with the obliquus capitis superior muscle.

The anterior rectus capitis, lateral rectus capitis, and obliquus capitis superior muscles belong systematically to the deep neck muscles, that is to the anterior part of the suboccipital musculature. Anatomically, however, they have to be considered as the continuation of the intertransverse muscles to the occiput, which again is supported by clinical experience with the SRS. Embryonically, the occiput represents a group of fused occipital vertebrae. Because of this, these three short suboccipital muscles are treated together with their corresponding intertransverse muscles. Thus, spondylogenically abbreviated, one deals with the myotenones C_0–C_1.

Intertransverse muscles of the thoracic region: They exist between T_2 and T_{10}, probably as the intertransverse ligament only.

Intertransverse muscles of the lumbar region: *The medial lumbar intertransverse muscles and the lateral lumbar intertransverse muscles.*

The posterior cervical intertransverse muscles, the thoracic intertransverse muscles, and the medial lumbar intertransverse muscles are considered one continuous and anatomical unit, which has been divided into the three muscle groups only as a result of their course through different anatomical regions with their respective local characteristics. In the cervical region they are found to overlap into the thoracic region, where, however, they are present mostly as ligaments. They are found as muscles again in the lumbar region. As a consequence of their division into the three distinct groups these muscles are presented in three different tables even though they belong systematically together. This is similar to the multifidus muscle, which consists of different segments also.

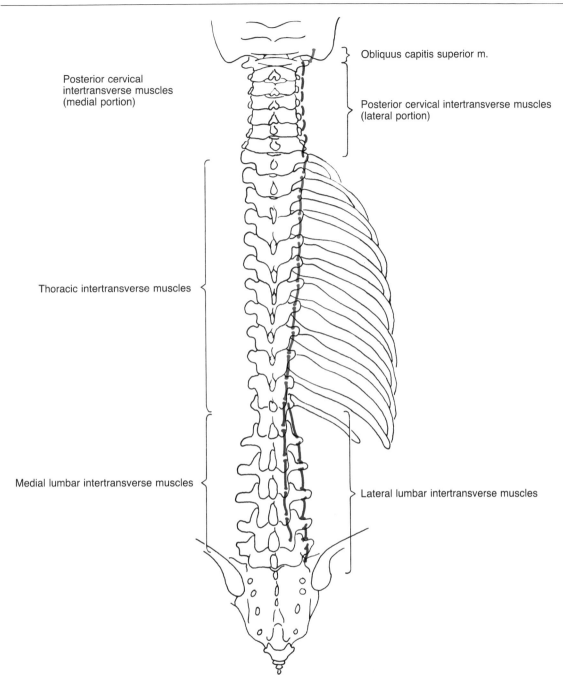

Obliquus capitis superior m.

Posterior cervical intertransverse muscles (lateral portion)

Posterior cervical intertransverse muscles (medial portion)

Thoracic intertransverse muscles

Medial lumbar intertransverse muscles

Lateral lumbar intertransverse muscles

Fig. **70**. Schematic representation of the intertransverse muscles.

7.2.1. Anterior Cervical Intertransverse Muscles

Origins and insertions: These short muscles are positioned between the anterior tubercles of the transverse processes of the cervical vertebrae. The most superior muscle lies between C_1 and C_2, the most inferior one lies between C_6 and C_7 (Fig. **71**).

Course and relations: With the exception of the first, all anterior cervical intertransverse muscles are covered at the anterior cervical spine by the longus colli and longus capitis muscle. Posteriorly, they are in proximity to the vertebral vessels. Anteriorly, they are close to the carotid artery.

Innervation: anterior rami of the corresponding spinal nerves.

Function: lateral flexion of the cervical spine, which is more of static than dynamic importance.

Palpatory technique: The anterior cervical intertransverse muscles lie practically behind the carotid artery. The anterior tubercles can be palpated anteriorly with the finger used for palpation pressing deeply at the medial margin of the sternocleidomastoid muscle and pushing the carotid artery medially. The palpatory direction for the origins and insertions is the same as the muscle direction. Caution is necessary with the carotid sinus at the C_4 level (see Fig. **51**, the cross-section for the cervical spine).

When the fingertip is placed between the two respective anterior tubercles, increased sensibility is evident. When changing the direction of the palpatory force appropriately, the tendinosis pain appears very distinctly.

7.2.2. Rectus Capitis Anterior Muscle

Origin: as a thin tendon from the lateral mass of the atlas (Fig. **71**).

Insertion: the basilar part of the occipital bone; starting about 6 to 8 mm distant from the pharyngeal tubercle and ending in front of the hypoglossal canal (Fig. **72**).

Course and relations: The rectus capitis anterior muscle lies in the immediate superior continuation of the first anterior cervical intertransverse muscle. The internal carotid artery, ascending pharyngeal artery, and the superior cervical (thyroid) ganglion of the sympathetic nervous system cross the anterior surface of the muscle laterally. At the lateral margin, the hypoglossal nerve appears superiorly. The posterior surface of the muscle lies next to the atlanto-occipital joint.

Innervation: ventral rami of C_1.

Function: bilateral contraction results in flexion of the head, and unilateral contraction results in lateral bending of the head to the side of the contracted muscle.

Palpatory technique: Due to its location, palpation is practically impossible.

SRS correlation: The anterior cervical intertransverse muscles along with the anterior rectus capitis muscle belong spondylogenically to C_1–C_7 in opposite sequence, however (see table). They frequently are involved in the spondylogenic event and can cause persistent unyielding relapse tendencies, especially in the central cervical spine, where the myotendinosis and the corresponding irritational zone meet on almost the exact same level, which in turn can lead to new abnormal positions or to the maintenance of the former abnormal position.

Spine	SRS Correlation			
C₀				
C₁	C₆	C₇		
C₂	C₅	C₆		
C₃	C₄	C₅		
C₄	C₃	C₄		
C₅	C₂	C₃		
C₆	C₁	C₂		
C₇	C₀	C₁		
T₁				
T₂				
T₃				
T₄				
T₅				
T₆				
T₇				
T₈				
T₉				
T₁₀				
T₁₁				
T₁₂				
L₁				
L₂				
L₃				
L₄				
L₅				
S₁				
S₂				
S₃				

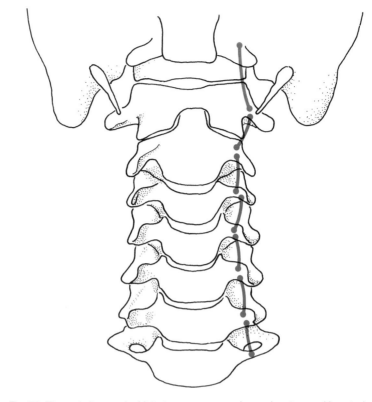

Fig. **71**. The anterior cervical intertransverse muscles and rectus capitis anterior muscle. Cervical spine, anterior view.

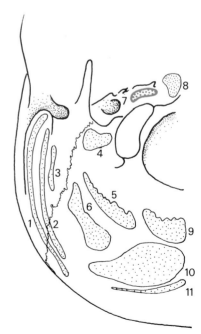

Fig. **72**. Muscle origins and insertions at the occiput.

1: Sternocleidomastoid m
2: Splenius capitis m
3: Longissimus capitis m
4: Rectus capitis lateralis m
5: Rectus capitis posterior major m
6: Obliquus capitis superior m
7: Rectus capitis anterior m
8: Longus capitis m
9: Rectus capitis posterior minor m
10: Semispinalis capitis m
11: Trapezius m

7.2.3. Posterior Cervical Intertransverse Muscles (Lateral Portion)

Origins and insertions: The muscles are fixed between the posterior tubercles of the cervical transverse processes. The most superior muscle lies between C_1 and C_2, the one most inferior, between C_6 and C_7. Further inferior, these muscles turn into the first levator costae muscle, which extends from the posterior margin of the first rib (the center of the neck to the costal tuberosity) to the posterior tuberosity of the transverse process of C_7 (Fig. **73**).

Course and relations: Posteriorly, they are almost fused with the medial portion of the posterior cervical intertransverse muscles. Posterolaterally, they lie next to the iliocostalis cervicis muscle ($C_{3(4)}$–C_6) and the longissimus cervicis muscle ($C_{1(2)}$–C_5).

Innervation: ventral rami of the corresponding spinal nerves.

Function: lateral flexion of the cervical vertebrae to the side of the contracted muscle.

Palpatory technique: The fingers press behind the sternocleidomastoid muscle on the posterior tubercles of the transverse processes. Differential diagnosis distinguishing between other muscles that attach here is not simple. The origins and insertions are examined according to the fiber direction of the muscle (compare Fig. **57** the cross sectional of the cervical spine). The procedure is analogous to that of the anterior cervical intertransverse muscles. Differentiation from the medial portion of the posterior cervical transverse muscles can prove to be difficult in this small area.

7.2.4. Rectus Capitis Lateralis Muscle

Origin: superior surface of the transverse process of the atlas, not including its posterior tubercle.

Insertion: lateral portion of the occipital bone reaching the center of the jugular foramen.

Course and relations: The rectus capitis lateralis muscle joins the posterior cervical intertransverse muscles (lateral portion), becoming their most superior member. Its medial surface borders on the ventral ramus of the first cervical nerve, while laterally the muscle adjoins to the posterior belly of the digastric muscle and the trunk of the facial nerve.

Innervation: ventral rami of C_1.

Function: lateral bending (lateralflexion) of the head.

Palpatory technique: One palpates around the transverse process of the atlas from a posteroinferior direction. To obtain contact with the occiput, one applies pressure, anteriorly. Consequently, the fingertip is between the atlas and the occiput and light pressure is exerted on the muscular insertions according to their directions.

Despite the close anatomical arrangement, the posterior cervical intertransverse muscles (lateral portion) and the rectus capitis lateralis muscle can be correlated with the thoracic and lumbar areas of the spine, whereas the anterior cervical intertransverse muscles cannot (see table). They frequently participate in the spondylogenic event.

Spine	SRS Correlation			
C_0				
C_1				
C_2				
C_3				
C_4				
C_5				
C_6				
C_7				
T_1				
T_2				
T_3				
T_4				
T_5				
T_6				
T_7	Posterior cervical intertransverse muscles (lateral portion)			
T_8				
T_9	C_6	C_7		
T_{10}	C_5	C_6		
T_{11}	C_4	C_5		
T_{12}	C_3	C_4		
L_1	C_2	C_3		
L_2	C_1	C_2		
L_3	Rectus capitis lateralis m			
	C_0	C_1		
L_4				
L_5				
S_1				
S_2				
S_3				

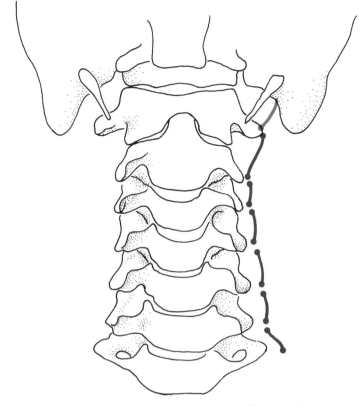

Fig. **73**. Posterior cervical intertransverse muscles (lateral portion) and lateral rectus capitis muscle. Cervical spine, anterior view.

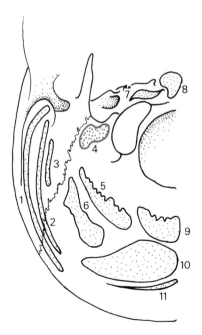

Fig. **74**. Muscle attachments at the occiput.

1: Sternocleidomastoid m
2: Splenius capitis m
3: Longissimus capitis m
4: Rectus capitis lateralis m
5: Rectus capitis posterior major m
6: Obliquus capitis superior m
7: Rectus capitis anterior m
8: Longus capitis m
9: Rectus capitis posterior minor m
10: Semispinalis capitis m
11: Trapezius m.

Fig. **75**. Suboccipital musculature.
1: Obliquus capitis inferior m
2: Obliquus capitis superior m
3: Rectus capitis posterior major m
4: Rectus capitis posterior minor m

7.2.5. Rectus Capitis Posterior Major Muscle

Origin: The rectus capitis posterior major muscle arises by a pointed tendinous origin from a narrow sagittal region on the lateral and superior half of the spinous process of the axis. The thick muscle belly takes on a triangular shape, with its muscle bundles spreading toward the skull. In this arrangement, the muscle fibers are twisted so that those bundles originating most anteriorly have their insertion medially (Fig. **75**).

Insertion: lateral half of the inferior nuchal line (Fig. **76**).

Course and relations: The rectus capitis posterior major muscle courses from its origin obliquely and superolaterally to the occiput and is primarily superimposed by the trapezius muscle (descending portion) and the semispinalis capitis muscle.

Innervation: dorsal rami of the spinal nerves C_1 and C_2.

Function: Bilateral contraction results in extension of the head, and unilateral contraction results in lateral bending to the side of the contracted muscle.

Palpatory technique: The muscle can easily be palpated. Starting from the mastoid process, the finger presses deeply under the semispinalis capitis muscle. The fleshy insertion presents itself in a region of 1×0.5 cm below the lateral third of inferior nuchal line. The lateral portion of the insertion is covered by the obliquus capitis superior muscle, and the medial portion is covered by the lateral part of the semispinalis capitis muscle. Palpation of the origin is according to the anatomical position. The palpatory direction is from superomedial to inferolateral.

SRS correlation: The whole rectus capitis posterior major muscle represents a single myotenone and is correlated with S_1.

Remarks: Myotendinosis of the rectus capitis posterior major muscle may influence the mechanics of the occipital-atlanto-axial joints via its origin at the spinous process of C_2.

7.2.6. Rectus Capitis Posterior Minor Muscle

Origin: tuberosity on the posterior arch of the atlas (Fig. **77**).

Insertion: between the medial third of the lower nuchal line and the external margin of the occiput (Fig. **78**).

Course and relations: superimposed mainly by the trapezius muscle (descending portion) and the semispinalis capitis muscle (medial portions).

Innervation: dorsal rami of the spinal nerves C_1 and C_2.

Function: Bilateral contraction results in extension of the head, and unilateral contraction results in lateral bending to the side of the contracted muscle. Due to its short leverage, however, the function of this muscle is of theoretical value only. The main function of this muscle is that of posture and stabilization of the occipitocervical junction.

Palpatory technique: About 2 cm below the external occipital protuberance, the finger used for palpation presses deeply between the two semispinalis capitis muscles. Palpatory direction is inferiorly, going from medial to lateral. Palpation of the origin at the posterior tuberosity of the atlas is according to its anatomical location.

SRS correlation: This occipital muscle also represents one singly myotenone, which is correlated with L_5.

Remarks: Myotendinotic changes in the rectus capitis posterior minor muscle can influence the normal physiological motion in the atlanto-occipital joints.

Spine	SRS Correlation			
C_0				
C_1				
C_2				
C_3				
C_4				
C_5				
C_6				
C_7				
T_1				
T_2				
T_3				
T_4				
T_5				
T_6				
T_7				
T_8				
T_9				
T_{10}				
T_{11}				
T_{12}				
L_1				
L_2				
L_3			Rectus capitis posterior minor m	
L_4	Rectus capitis posterior major m			
L_5			C_0	C_1
S_1	C_0	C_2		
S_2				
S_3				

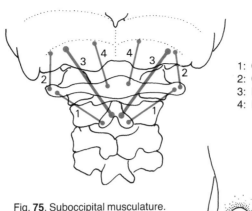

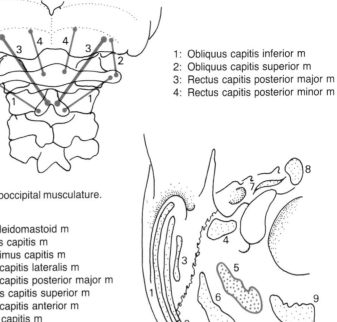

Fig. **75**. Suboccipital musculature.

1: Obliquus capitis inferior m
2: Obliquus capitis superior m
3: Rectus capitis posterior major m
4: Rectus capitis posterior minor m

1: Sternocleidomastoid m
2: Splenius capitis m
3: Longissimus capitis m
4: Rectus capitis lateralis m
5: Rectus capitis posterior major m
6: Obliquus capitis superior m
7: Rectus capitis anterior m
8: Longus capitis m
9: Rectus capitis posterior minor m
10: Semispinalis capitis m
11: Trapezius m

Fig. **76**. Muscle attachments at the occiput.

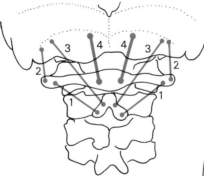

Fig. **77**. Suboccipital musculature.

1: Obliquus capitis inferior m
2: Obliquus capitis superior m
3: Rectus capitis posterior major m
4: Rectus capitis posterior minor m

1: Sternocleidomastoid m
2: Splenius capitis m
3: Longissimus capitis m
4: Rectus capitis lateralis m
5: Rectus capitis posterior major m
6: Obliquus capitis superior m
7: Rectus capitis anterior m
8: Longus capitis m
9: Rectus capitis posterior minor m
10: Semispinalis capitis m
11: Trapezius m

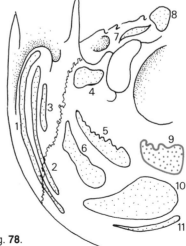

Fig. **78**.
Muscle attachments at the occiput.

7.2.7. Posterior Cervical Intertransverse Muscles (Medial Portion)

Origins and insertions: The medial portion of the posterior cervical intertransverse muscles, like the lateral portion of the posterior cervical intertransverse muscles extends between the posterior tuberosities of the spinous processes, although somewhat more posteriorly. The most superior segments are between C_2 and C_1 (at the transverse process of C_1 between the obliquus capitis inferior muscle and the splenius cervicis muscle), and the most inferior portion is located between rib I and C_7 (inferior surface of the posterior tubercle) (Figs. 79, 80).

Course and relations: practically the same as the lateral portion of the posterior cervical intertransverse muscles.

Innervation: dorsal rami of the cervical nerves C_2–C_7.

Function: lateral flexion of the vertebrae to the side of the contracted muscle.

Palpatory technique: Palpation is the same as for the lateral portion of the posterior cervical intertransverse muscles. Palpatory differential diagnosis can be difficult in such a small region, but can become evident from the overall presentation of the SRS.

7.2.8. Obliquus Capitis Superior Muscle

Origin: This muscle arises by thick tendinous fibers from the posterior corner and the lateral segment of the transverse process of C_1 (Fig. 81).

Insertion: superior to the lateral third of the inferior nuchal line.

Innervation: dorsal rami of C_1.

Function: Bilateral contraction results in extension of the head, and unilateral contraction results in lateral bending of the head to the side of the contracted muscle.

Palpatory technique: The origin is palpated quite inferiorly below the most lateral insertion of the semispinalis capitis muscle (about 3 cm lateral to the external occipital protuberance). The origin is palpated superoposteriorly in the direction of the tip of the transverse process of the atlas.

SRS correlation: The posterior cervical intertransverse muscles and the obliquus capitis superior muscle play an important role in the spondylogenic event. The correlation can be seen from the table. Even though the obliquus capitis superior muscle belongs anatomically to the posterior cervical intertransverse muscle group, it is spondylogenically and reflexogenically correlated with the S_3 segment.

7.2.9. Obliquus Capitis Inferior Muscle

Origin: anteriorly between the apex of the spinous process of the axis, the arch.

Insertion: inferior and posterior surface of the transverse process of the atlas reaching the root of its posterior part.

Course and relations: See Fig. 82.

Innervation: dorsal rami of the spinal nerves C_1 and C_2.

Function: rotation of the head to the side of the contracted muscle.

Palpatory technique: The origin is palpated laterally at the spinous process of C_2 according to the direction of the muscle fibers. The insertion at the transverse process of the atlas, is palpated medioinferiorly. The correct palpatory depth has to be assured for both the origin and the insertion. It is very difficult to distinguish the insertion tendinosis from the zone of irritation. Myotendinotic changes in the muscle belly appear in the suboccipital soft tissue as a perpendicular, laterosuperiorly directed spindle.

SRS correlation: The whole muscle is correlated as one single myotenone with S_2 (see table).

Spine	SRS Correlation			
C_0				
C_1				
C_2				
C_3				
C_4				
C_5				
C_6				
C_7				
T_1				
T_2				
T_3				
T_4	Obliquus capitis inferior m			
T_5				
T_6	C_2	C_1		
T_7				
T_8	Obliquus capitis superior m		Posterior cervical intertrans-verse muscles	
T_9				
T_{10}	C_0	C_1		
T_{11}			C_1	C_2
T_{12}			C_2	C_3
L_1			C_3	C_4
L_2			C_4	C_5
L_3			C_5	C_6
L_4			C_6	C_7
L_5			C_7	T_1
S_1				
S_2				
S_3				

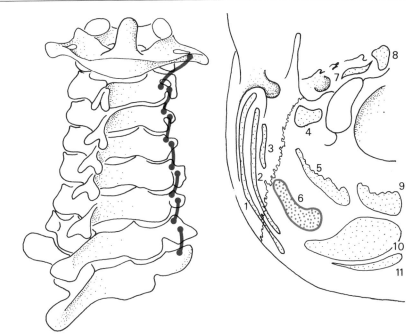

Fig. **79**. Posterior cervical intertransverse muscles (medial portion).

Fig. **80**. Muscle attachments at the occiput.

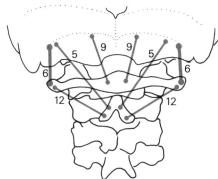

Fig. **81**. Suboccipital muscles.

1: Sternocleidomastoid m
2: Splenius capitis m
3: Longissimus capitis m
4: Rectus capitis lateralis m
5: Rectus capitis posterior major m
6: Obliquus capitis superior m
7: Rectus capitis anterior m
8: Longus capitis m
9: Rectus capitis posterior minor m
10: Semispinalis capitis m
11: Trapezius m
12: Obliquus capitis inferior m

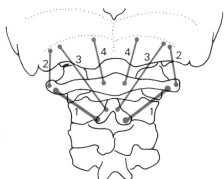

1: Inferior obliquus capitis m
2: Superior obliquus capitis m
3: Rectus capitis posterior major m
4: Rectus capitis posterior minor m

Fig. **82**. Suboccipital muscles.

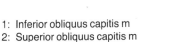

7.2.10. Thoracic Intertransverse Muscles

Three pairs of these muscles are normally present, the rest being either ligamentous or absorbed in the long musculature, mainly the longissimus muscle.

Origin and insertion: These are short muscles, which are principally located between the individual transverse processes, from the inferior margin of the superior thoracic transverse process to the superior border of the inferior thoracic transverse process. The last muscle often divides into two portions, arising from the inferior surface of the transverse process of T_{11} and reaching the mamillary and accessory processes of T_{12} (Fig. **83**).

This bifurcation can sometimes continue into the lumbar spinal region. Thus, the continuation of the thoracic intertransverse muscles into the lumbar spinal region is formed by the medial lumbar intertransverse muscles, which in turn are divided into a medial and lateral portion. This is of no relevance to the diagnosis, however.

Course and relations: These muscles belong to the deep and short autochthonous musculature and therefore lie beneath the rest of the muscles. At the last thoracic and lumbar vertebrae, they nestle between the longissimus muscle (lateral) and the multifidus muscle, (medioposterior).

Innervation: dorsal rami of the segmental nerves.

Function: lateral flexion of the corresponding vertebrae.

Palpatory technique: Palpation of these small and deep spondylogenic units in the thoracic region and especially the differentiation from neighboring tendinoses are very difficult. The fingertip is placed over the origin and insertion on the skeleton and then the halfway point is determined, from which only the direction of the palpatory pressure is changed: along the muscle belly in the direction of the origin tendinosis and in the opposite direction to the insertion tendinosis!

SRS correlation: From clinical experience, it is also known that in the area of the so-called non-developed posterior thoracic intertransverse muscles a regular myotendinosis can be found. This shows that the phenomenon of myotendinosis with its clinical correlation does not necessarily require the presence of real muscle tissue. The spondylogenic correlation can be seen in the following table.

Spine	SRS Correlation			
C_0			T_1	T_2
C_1			T_2	T_3
C_2			T_3	T_4
C_3			T_4	T_5
C_4			T_5	T_6
C_5			T_6	T_7
C_6			T_7	T_8
C_7			T_8	T_9
T_1			T_9	T_{10}
T_2			T_{10}	T_{11}
T_3			T_{11}	T_{12}
T_4			T_{12}	L_1
T_5				
T_6				
T_7				
T_8				
T_9				
T_{10}				
T_{11}				
T_{12}				
L_1				
L_2				
L_3				
L_4				
L_5				
S_1				
S_2				
S_3				

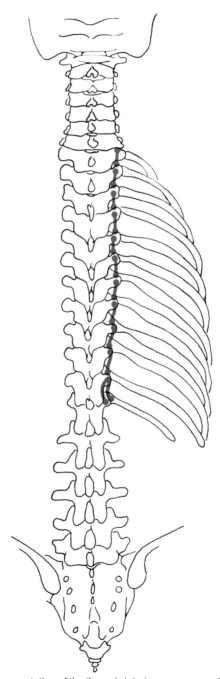

Fig. **83**. Schematic representation of the thoracic intertransverse muscles.

7.2.11. Medial Lumbar Intertransverse Muscles

The medial lumbar intertransverse muscles can exist as one single unit or they can be divided into a medial and lateral portion, starting from their insertions (compare thoracic intertransverse muscles) (Figs. **84, 85**).

Origin: Inferior margin of the accessory process, tendinous arch to the inferior border of the mamillary process (nerve exit, dorsal ramus of the spinal nerves; Fig. **85**).

Insertion: between the superior edge of the adjoining mamillary process anteriorly and the root of the costal process and the superior edge of the accessory process. It normally does not reach below L_5.

Course and relations: The sagittally oriented muscle belly lies in the deep muscle layer between the longissimus muscle (lateral) and the multifidus muscle (medioposterior and dorsal).

Innervation: dorsal rami of the spinal nerves.

Palpatory technique: Palpation of this muscle is difficult due to its close proximity to the transversospinal system and is thus only possible in isolated circumstances. The muscle often causes paravertebral lumbar pain. Considering the anatomical arrangement, the general principles of the palpatory technique apply here as well.

SRS correlation: See table.

7.2.12. Lateral Lumbar Intertransverse Muscles

Origin: the superior margin of the costal process, from the tip to its root, with exit of the dorsal ramus of the spinal nerves. The most inferior muscle originates at the lateral mass of S_1 (Fig. **86**).

Insertion: The muscle located most superiorly inserts at the lateral tubercle of T_{12} and the lumbocostal ligament; all others insert at the inferior border, reaching to the tip of the costal process.

Innervation: dorsal rami of the spinal nerves.

Function: lateral flexion of the vertebra involved to the side of the contracted muscle.

Palpatory technique: Myotendinosis of the lateral lumbar intertransverse muscles must be distinguished from the corresponding segmental zones of irritation by provocative testing (compare page 56).

It is best to palpate from both sides simultaneously, whereby both thumbs reach around and below the sacrospinal system and do not press directly on the tip of the costal processes, but rather between the two costal processes in order to palpate them inferiorly and superiorly.

SRS correlation: The lateral lumbar intertransverse muscles are associated with the upper thoracic spine (see table). They often are involved in the SRS event and palpatory access is usually easy. Thus, they are of practical importance for the beginner both for the diagnosis and therapy.

Remarks: The quadratus lumbar muscle and the longissimus lumbar muscle must be differentiated diagnostically from each other.

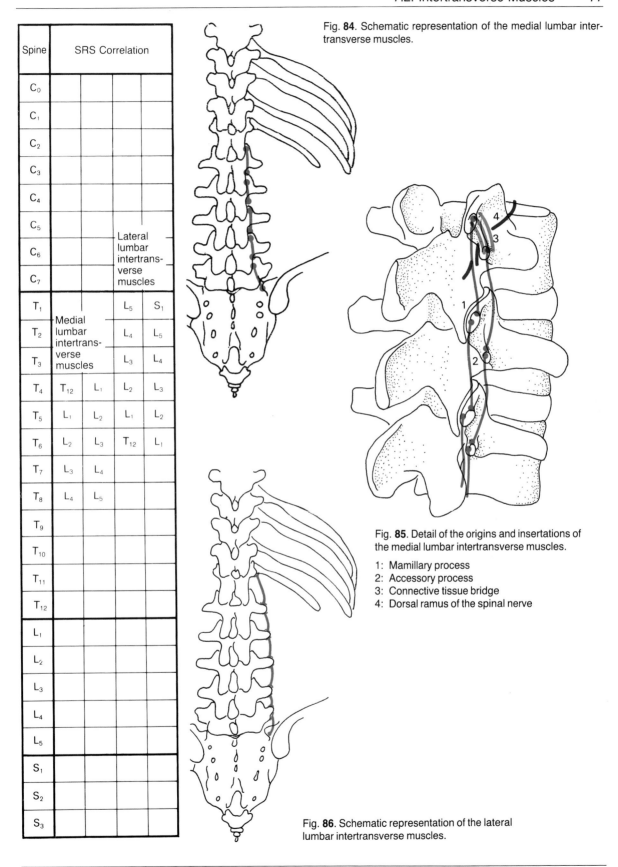

Spine	SRS Correlation			
C_0				
C_1				
C_2				
C_3				
C_4				
C_5			Lateral lumbar intertrans- verse muscles	
C_6				
C_7				
T_1	Medial lumbar intertrans- verse muscles		L_5	S_1
T_2			L_4	L_5
T_3			L_3	L_4
T_4	T_{12}	L_1	L_2	L_3
T_5	L_1	L_2	L_1	L_2
T_6	L_2	L_3	T_{12}	L_1
T_7	L_3	L_4		
T_8	L_4	L_5		
T_9				
T_{10}				
T_{11}				
T_{12}				
L_1				
L_2				
L_3				
L_4				
L_5				
S_1				
S_2				
S_3				

Fig. **84**. Schematic representation of the medial lumbar intertransverse muscles.

Fig. **85**. Detail of the origins and insertions of the medial lumbar intertransverse muscles.

1: Mamillary process
2: Accessory process
3: Connective tissue bridge
4: Dorsal ramus of the spinal nerve

Fig. **86**. Schematic representation of the lateral lumbar intertransverse muscles.

7.3. Longus Colli Muscle

Origin: See Figures **87** and **88**.

Superior portion: the anterior tubercle and anterior surface of the transverse processes.

Inferior portion: lateral side of the vertebral bodies of C_5–C_7 and the anterolateral portion of the vertebral bodies of T_1–T_3 (strong, always).

Insertion:

Superior portion: the tubercle on the anterior arch of the atlas and vertebral bodies of C_2–C_4, immediately next to the longitudinal ligament.

Inferior portion: the most inferior side on the anterior surface of the transverse processes of C_5–C_7.

Function: Bilateral contraction results in flexion of the cervical spine, and unilateral contraction results in lateral bending of the head to the side of the contracted muscle.

Innervation: ventral rami of the spinal nervs C_2–C_6.

Palpatory technique: Origin tendinosis can be palpated superomedially after having moved the sternocleidomastoid muscle aside.

The origins of the inferior portion cannot be palpated due to the position and course of the scalene muscles. The insertion at C_1 can be palpated inferiorly. This may be confused with the zone of irritation of C_1. To reach the insertions at C_2–C_4, the finger presses deeply between the sternocleidomastoid muscle and the pharynx. Because of the anatomical location and relation to the pharynx palpation is difficult and thus not always useful for diagnosis.

SRS correlation: See Figure **88** and the table. Due to its reflexogenic correlation to the upper thoracic spine, the longus colli muscle takes part in the spondylogenic event and can cause an anteriorly abnormal position of a cervical vertebra.

One should observe the response of the zone of irritation upon provocative testing of the cervical spine.

7.4. Longus Colli and Longus Capitis Muscles

Origin: with four projections from the anterior tubercles of the transverse processes of C_3–C_6, between the origins of the longus colli muscle and anterior scalene muscle.

Insertion: at the pharyngeal tubercle, about one-half of a finger width from the anterior condyle at the occiput, the basilar part of the occipital bone.

Innervation: ventral rami of C_1–C_3.

Function: flexion of the head.

Palpatory technique: Similar to the longus colli muscle, the origins are palpated from a superior direction. The insertion at the occiput cannot be easily palpated. To test for possible myotendinosis in the muscle belly the orientation is best at the C_3 level. The recognition of myotendinosis in the longus system is of therapeutic importance. Myotendinosis is responsible for the anterior component of the abnormal position, which is rather seldom, however.

SRS correlation: See Figure **88** and the table.

Spine	SRS Correlation			
C_0				
C_1				
C_2				
C_3				
C_4				
C_5				
C_6				
C_7			Longus capitis m	
T_1	Longus colli m			C_6
T_2	C_3	C_1		C_5
T_3	C_4	C_2		C_4
T_4	C_5	C_3		C_3
T_5	C_6	C_4		
T_6				
T_7				
T_8	T_1	C_5		
T_9	T_2	C_6		
T_{10}	T_3	C_7		
T_{11}				
T_{12}				
L_1				
L_2				
L_3				
L_4				
L_5				
S_1				
S_2				
S_3				

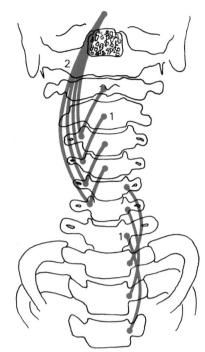

Fig. **87**. Longi colli and capitis muscles.

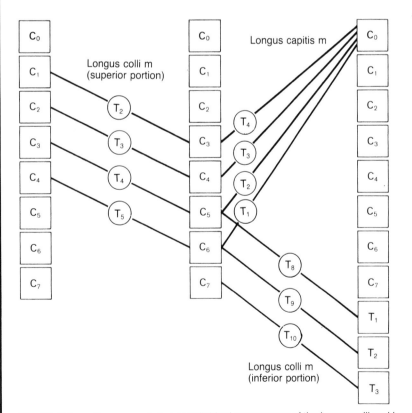

Fig. **88**. Schematic representation of individual myotenones of the longus colli and longus capitis muscles and their spondylogenic correlation.

7.5.   Rotatores Breves and Longi Muscles

Origin: Cervical region, from the posterior boundary of the superior articular process. Thoracic region, from the transverse process (medial portions, see diagram). Lumbar region, from the mamillary process.

Insertion: cervical region at the inferolateral margin of the spinous processes of the next one or two vertebrae above. Thoracic and lumbar regions at the vertebral arch (Fig. **89**).

Course and relations: These muscles course above the posteromedial boundary of the upper apophyseal joints (cervical spine). The breves muscles are almost horizontal, whereas the longi muscles are angled superomedially (Fig. **90**).

Innervation: dorsal rami of the corresponding segmental nerves.

Function: Bilateral contraction results in extension of the superior vertebra, and unilateral contraction results in rotation of the superior vertebra to the other side.

Palpatory technique: The insertions are palpated according to the fiber direction of the muscle, from lateral to medial whereas the origins are palpated from the medial to the lateral. The muscle is palpated perpendicularly in the direction of the fibers. Even though of small size, the rotatores muscles can be detected palpatorily, since they lie directly above the hard skeleton with minimal amounts of soft tissue intervening. In order to determine whether myotendinosis is present, the fingertip must be introduced carefully and slowly into the spinotransverse vertebral groove so as finally to reach definite contact with the bones of the articulating processes (cervical spine, thoracic spine) or the vertebral arches of the laminae (lumbar spine).

SRS correlation: In contrast to the anatomical unit the spondylogenic unit is represented as the myotenone depicted in Figure **91**. In practice one finds with an abnormal position of L_3 (zone of irritation), for instance, a myotendinosis or tendinosis (latent zone) in the spondylogenically associated myotenone at the T_7, T_8, or T_9 levels: at the T_7 level, at the insertion at the vertebral arch, and at T_8 and T_9 levels, at the origin on the transverse process (see table). The tendinoses at the transverse processes are accompanied by corresponding segmental zones of irritations, especially in the thoracic spine region.

Remarks: The distinction between the rotatores longi and breves muscles dates back to the nomenclature of Basle. Some books incorrectly correlate the rotatores longi and breves muscles with the multifidus muscle and designate them as its deepest layer.

Spine	SRS Correlation		
C_0	T_10	T_11	T_12
C_1	T_11	T_12	L_1
C_2	T_12	L_1	L_2
C_3	L_1	L_2	L_3
C_4	L_2	L_3	L_4
C_5	L_3	L_4	L_5
C_6	L_4	L_5	S_1
C_7	L_5	S_1	S_2
T_1		C_2	C_3
T_2	C_1	C_2	C_3
T_3	C_2	C_3	C_4
T_4	C_3	C_4	C_5
T_5	C_4	C_5	C_6
T_6	C_5	C_6	C_7
T_7	C_6	C_7	T_1
T_8	C_7	T_1	T_2
T_9	T_1	T_2	T_3
T_10	T_2	T_3	T_4
T_11	T_3	T_4	T_5
T_12	T_4	T_5	T_6
L_1	T_5	T_6	T_7
L_2	T_6	T_7	T_8
L_3	T_7	T_8	T_9
L_4	T_8	T_9	T_10
L_5	T_9	T_10	T_11
S_1	T_10	T_11	T_12
S_2	T_11	T_12	L_1
S_3	T_12	L_1	L_2

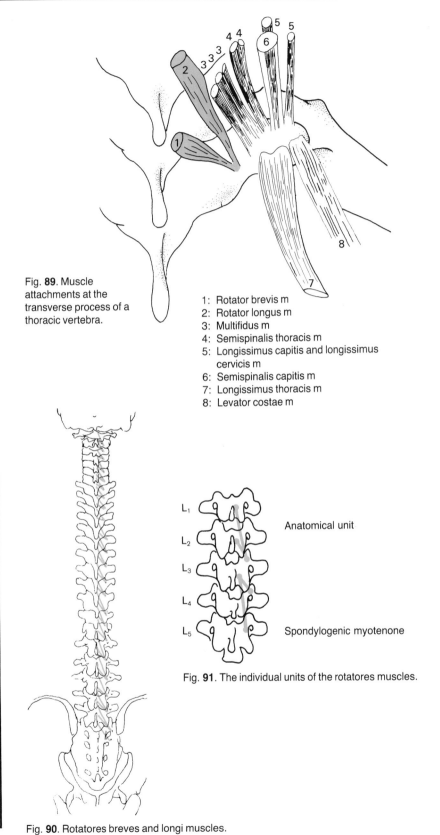

Fig. **89**. Muscle attachments at the transverse process of a thoracic vertebra.

1: Rotator brevis m
2: Rotator longus m
3: Multifidus m
4: Semispinalis thoracis m
5: Longissimus capitis and longissimus cervicis m
6: Semispinalis capitis m
7: Longissimus thoracis m
8: Levator costae m

Anatomical unit

Spondylogenic myotenone

Fig. **91**. The individual units of the rotatores muscles.

Fig. **90**. Rotatores breves and longi muscles.

7.6.   Multifidus Muscle

With the origins of the multifidus muscles extending from $C_{4(5)}$ to S_4, and the insertions from C_2 to L_5, the multifidus muscle has quite a complicated structure. Yet, it is possible to anatomically divide this muscle into four different groups (Virchow): the cervical, the upper thoracic, the lower thoracic, and the lumbar (Fig. **92**).

Cervical Group (from T_1 to C_2):

Origin: from the posterior border of the inferior articular process of the cervical spine, whereby the origins can reach the deep posterior surface of the vertebral arch. The origin at T_1 is located at the superior border of the transverse process up to the root.

Insertion: in the ipsilateral tips of the bifurcated cervical spinous processes up to C_2, where they occupy almost the entire inferior border.

Upper Thoracic Group (from T_7 to T_1):

Origin: transverse processes of T_2–T_6 (Fig. **89**).

Insertion: inferior margins of the spinous processes up to C_5.

Lower Thoracic Group (from L_1 to T_7):

Origin: similar to the upper thoracic portion; the origins extend from the arch to the neck of the transverse process.

Insertion: inferior margins of the spinous processes from the tip to the root.

Lumbar Group (from S_4 to L_1):

Origin: very complicated, from the posterior sacrum to S_4, from the median sacral crest at S_3–S_4, then laterally from the lateral sacral crest and the posterior sacroiliac ligaments to the posterior end of the iliac crest. In the lower lumbar region from the mamillary processes.

Insertion: inferior margins of all lumbar and thoracic spinous processes to T_7.

Course and relations: The fasciculi of this muscle draw out from their origin in the mediosuperior direction to the spinous process. Its structure is very complicated in the cervical and lumbar spine regions. Its muscle mass fills the groove between the transverse and spinous processes. It covers the rotatores muscles and vertebral arches, is positioned laterally to the interspinales muscles, and is beneath the semispinalis muscle. In the lumbosacral region, it is covered by the muscle belly and the origin and aponeurosis of the longissimus thoracis muscle.

Innervation: the medial branches of the dorsal rami of the spinal nerves C_3–L_5.

Function: Bilateral contraction results in extension of the vertebral column, and unilateral contraction results in rotation of the vertebral column to the opposite side.

Palpatory technique: Like the rotatores muscle, the multifidus muscle is difficult to palpate because of its deep location. In accordance with the direction of the muscle fibers, the origins are palpated in the mediosuperior direction and the insertion in the lateroinferior direction. To prevent confusion, the correct palpatory direction and palpatory depth must first be established and then sustained. In contrast to the anatomical arrangement, for palpation, the finger finds the insertion at the portion of the spinous process close to the arch. From the arrangement of the entire myotenone one can determine whether or not the muscle is a member of the multifidus group by using spondylogenic correlation with the appropriate zone of irritation four segments more superior than the uniform insertion area of tendinosis.

SRS correlation (see the table): The multifidus muscle very often participates in the spondylogenic event. Despite its deep location, it can easily be palpated (see before). With an L_4 abnormal position (zone of irritation) for instance, one palpates an origin tendinosis at the transverse process of T_{12}, and the insertion tendinoses according to the myotenone structure at the roots of the spinous processes of T_7–T_9 (Fig. **93**).

Remarks: The muscle fibers generally fan out from their origin in three fasciculi, resulting in three insertions, and thus creating a functional and spondylogenic unit three to five vertebral levels higher (the so-called myotenone) (Fig. **93**).

The portion of the muscle inserting at the spinous process of C_2 may consist of components from all origins of C_4 or C_3 to T_1.

Spine	SRS Correlation			
C_0	T_9	T_{10}	T_{11}	L_2
C_1	T_{10}	T_{11}	T_{12}	L_3
C_2	T_{11}	T_{12}	L_1	L_4
C_3	T_{12}	L_1	L_2	L_5
C_4	L_1	L_2	L_3	S_1
C_5	L_2	L_3	L_4	S_2
C_6	L_3	L_4	L_5	S_3
C_7	L_4	L_5		S_4
T_1	C_2			C_4
T_2	C_2			C_5
T_3	C_2	C_3		C_6
T_4	C_2	C_3	C_4	C_7
T_5	C_3	C_4	C_5	T_1
T_6	C_4	C_5	C_6	T_2
T_7	C_5	C_6	C_7	T_3
T_8	C_6	C_7	T_1	T_4
T_9	C_7	T_1	T_2	T_5
T_{10}	T_1	T_2	T_3	T_6
T_{11}	T_2	T_3	T_4	T_7
T_{12}	T_3	T_4	T_5	T_8
L_1	T_4	T_5	T_6	T_9
L_2	T_5	T_6	T_7	T_{10}
L_3	T_6	T_7	T_8	T_{11}
L_4	T_7	T_8	T_9	T_{12}
L_5	T_8	T_9	T_{10}	L_1
S_1	T_9	T_{10}	T_{11}	L_2
S_2	T_{10}	T_{11}	T_{12}	L_3
S_3	T_{11}	T_{12}	L_1	L_4

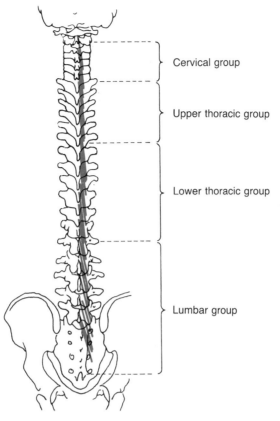

Cervical group

Upper thoracic group

Lower thoracic group

Lumbar group

Fig. **92**. Multifidus muscle.

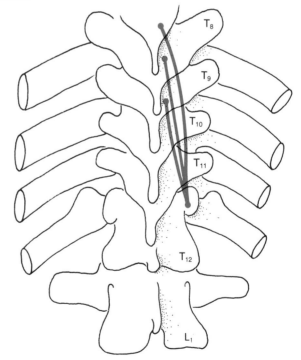

Fig. **93**. The multifidus myotenone; it can be palpated with a segmental dysfunction of L_4 (see SRS correlation).

7.7. Semispinalis Muscle

General remarks

This muscle is a flat, nonuniform mass, a system consisting of many fasciculi. The muscular units overlap superoinferiorly in a tile-roof manner. This characteristic feature of the transversospinal system, starting from the axis going inferiorly, is due to the fact that the muscle fibers arriving from the individual transverse processes cannot be associated with one single vertebra, but rather fan out into several portions. These individual portions then insert on different vertebrae, explaining the different lengths. For the long muscle segments (superficial), the direction of the fibers is almost vertical, whereas the short (deep) muscle portions run almost in a transverse direction (Fig. **94**).

7.7.1. Semispinalis Lumborum Muscle

Origin: This muscle arises by a strong fascia from the mamillary processes of S_1, L_5, and L_2; from the mamillary processes of L_1 and T_{12}, it arises directly.

Insertion: It inserts as long tendons at the inferior portions of those two spinous processes that are positioned six and seven segments superior to that vertebra from which the myotenone originates. The anatomical muscular unit of the semispinalis muscle described here is identical to the spondylogenic unit, the myotenone.

7.7.2. Semispinalis Thoracis and Cervicis Muscles

Origin: from the superior edge of the transverse process, that is, the thoracic portion from T_6–T_{10}, and the cervical region from T_2–T_5 (Fig. **95**).

Insertion: The structure of the myotenone remains the same, as described previously. The insertions are found at the spinous processes, which are six to seven segmental levels higher than the vertebra from which the myotenone originates. The insertion tendinosis is usually best developed in the medioposterior region (Fig. **95**).

Course and relations: All three semispinales muscles are positioned at the same level. The superior surface is covered by the longissimus muscle, the spinalis muscle, and partially the semispinalis capitis muscle. A thin connective tissue layer demarcates this muscle from the multifidus muscle below, which is important for palpation. Differentiation from the multifidus muscle is facilitated by the fact that the longest portions of the multifidus muscle skip two fewer vertebrae than the semispinalis muscle.

Innervation: dorsal rami of the spinal nerves.

Function: Bilateral contraction results in extension of the vertebral column, and unilateral contraction results in rotation of the vertebral column contralaterally.

Palpatory technique: Due to its frequent spondylogenic participation, exact palpation of the transversospinal system is extremely important. As a result of the close anatomical arrangement, one cannot distinguish at the mamillary or transverse process whether the origin tendinosis belongs to the semispinalis muscle, the multifidus muscle, or the rotatores muscles. Only when the attachment tendinoses are present in both directions is differentiation possible. The rotatores muscles pass from one vertebra to the next or the second next above (be aware of the difference between the anatomical and spondylogenic units). The multifidus muscle passes from one vertebra to the next third above and inserts via three fasciculi. The semispinalis muscle extends from one vertebra to the sixth above and inserts via two fasciculi. When we locate a painful superior margin of the mamillary bodies, we must palpate all seven spinous processes from their lateral aspect to the root in order to eliminate the rotatores muscles and the multifidus muscle.

The origin tendinosis is determined to belong to the semispinalis muscle when the insertion is on opposite poles and lies six to seven levels superior at the roots of the spinous process. The myotendinosis of the individual muscle fibers can normally be palpated as a thin matchlike band.

SRS correlation: The spondylogenic unit, the myotenone, is represented in Figure **96**. The 17 myotenones of the semispinalis muscle are correlated with segments C_0–T_9 (see table).

Spine	SRS Correlation			
C_0	T_{11}	T_{12}		S_1
C_1	T_{10}	T_{11}		L_5
C_2	T_9	T_{10}		L_4
C_3	T_8	T_9		L_3
C_4	T_7	T_8		L_2
C_5	T_6	T_7		L_1
C_6	T_5	T_6		T_{12}
C_7	T_4	T_5		T_{11}
T_1	T_3	T_4		T_{10}
T_2	T_2	T_3		T_9
T_3	T_1	T_2		T_8
T_4	C_7	T_1		T_7
T_5	C_6	C_7		T_6
T_6	C_5	C_6		T_5
T_7	C_4	C_5		T_4
T_8	C_3	C_4		T_3
T_9	C_2	C_3		T_2
T_{10}				
T_{11}				
T_{12}				
L_1				
L_2				
L_3				
L_4				
L_5				
S_1				
S_2				
S_3				

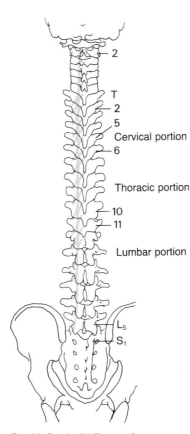

Cervical portion

Thoracic portion

Lumbar portion

Fig. **94**. Semispinalis muscle.

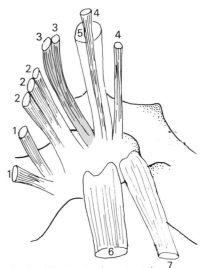

Fig. **95**. Muscle attachments at the transverse process of a thoracic vertebra.
1: Rotatores muscles
2: Multifidus m
3: Semispinalis cervicis m
4: Longissimus cervicis and capitis m
5: Semispinalis capitis m
6: Longissimus thoracis m
7: Levator costae m

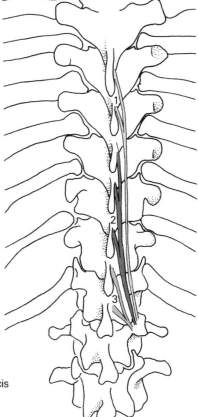

Fig. **96**.
1: Myotenone of the semispinalis thoracis muscle
2: Myotenone of the multifidus muscle
3: Rotatores longus and brevis muscles

7.7.3. **Semispinalis Capitis Muscle**

Origin: This muscle arises from the root of the transverse processes of C_3–C_6 (which is in close proximity to the insertions of the posterior scalene muscles, the levator scapulae muscle, the splenius cervicis muscle, the iliocostalis cervicis muscle, the longissimus cervicis muscle, the longissimus capitis muscle, and the posterior cervical intertransverse muscles). Further, it arises from the thick tip of the transverse processes of C_7, T_1–T_8 and posterosuperiorly from the planum nuchale (Fig. **97**).

Insertion: The semispinalis capitis muscle inserts in the planum nuchale of the occipital bone directly beside the midline. The insertion has a characteristic shape (see diagram) and lies between the superior and inferior nuchal lines. In the transverse direction it measures about 3 cm, in the sagittal direction, about 2 cm (Fig. **99**).

Course and relations: The semispinalis capitis muscles being lateral to the nuchal ligament, overlies the bifurcated spinous processes of the cervical spine, including C_7. Further inferiorly, it is imbedded superficially in a bony and ligamentous groove formed by the spinous processes, vertebral arches, apophyseal joints and transverse processes. In the thoracic region, it is situated lateral to the thoracic spinous processes. The muscle itself is flat and superficial in the medial neck portion. In the cervical region, it is covered by the splenius capitis muscle and the trapezius muscle only. The semispinalis capitis muscle covers the semispinalis cervicis muscle as well as a portion of the semispinalis thoracis muscle. As a result, when palpating one perceives the semispinalis capitis muscle as a round bundle. It borders the longissimus capitis muscle laterally (Fig. **98**).

Innervation: dorsal rami of the cervical nerves C_1–C_4.

Function: Bilateral contraction results in extension of the head and the cervical spine, and unilateral contraction results in rotation of the head and the cervical spine contralaterally.

Palpatory technique: The whole muscle mass is examined in the cervical region at the C_3 level, where the muscle has a cylindrical appearance. By palpating from medial to lateral (that is, perpendicular to the fiber direction), one can detect possible myotendinosis. When the semispinalis capitis muscle is palpated following an arch, one reaches the deep articular and transverse processes. The longissimus and cervicis muscles lie lateral to the finger being used for palpation. The tips of the transverse processes must be examined from the posterosuperior direction (if the direction of palpation is altered, one can confuse them with other muscles). When palpating, one should be aware of the close anatomical relationship between the tendinoses and the segmental zones of irritation. Thus, when the head is in a neutral position, the area of insertion is located at the inferior portion of the planum nuchale of the occipital bone. When the head is flexed, it rises and thus exposes its upper portions superiorly. This area of insertion is differentiated from other muscle insertions at the posterior occiput as a result of the cushioning effect of the soft tissue. The palpatory direction is from the inferior and can be followed to the lateral end (about 3.5 cm from the external occipital protuberance). At the thoracocervical junction, it is very difficult to palpate the myotenones that arise inferior to T_3. Here the muscle belly is simply a tendon in which the myotendinotic changes appear weakly.

SRS correlation:

1. Each origin of the semispinalis capitis muscle represents one individual myotenone.
2. Each of these myotendinoses is correlated with one particular SRS.
3. Each myotenone of the semispinalis capitis muscle belongs to that SRS, whose causative functional abnormal position (segmental dysfunction) is located eight vertebral levels more inferior ("rules of eight").

With an abnormal position of L_3, for instance, (zone of irritation), we find myotendinoses in its spondylogenically related myotenone, in this case at the transverse process of T_7 and furthermore at its insertion area at the occiput (see table and Fig. 99).

Remarks: The myotendinoses of T_5–T_6 demonstrate a special relationship to the greater occipital nerve. With myotendinosis, sensory disturbances in the field of innervation of the nerve can appear.

The semispinalis capitis muscle therefore represents to some degree a mirror image of the sacrospinal system and as such is often affected in the spondylogenic event.

Clinically, myotendinosis in the semispinalis capitis muscle can result in a persistent headache radiating from the occipital to the frontal areas.

Spine	SRS Correlation			
C_0				
C_1				
C_2				
C_3				
C_4				
C_5				
C_6				
C_7				
T_1				
T_2				
T_3				
T_4	C_3			
T_5	C_4			
T_6	C_5			
T_7	C_6			
T_8	C_7			
T_9	T_1			
T_{10}	T_2			
T_{11}	T_3			
T_{12}	T_4			
L_1	T_5			
L_2	T_6			
L_3	T_7			
L_4	T_8			
L_5				
S_1				
S_2				
S_3				

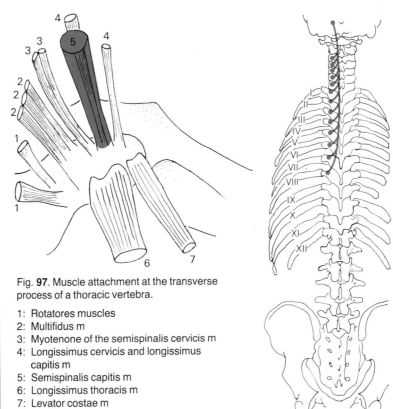

Fig. **97**. Muscle attachment at the transverse process of a thoracic vertebra.

1: Rotatores muscles
2: Multifidus m
3: Myotenone of the semispinalis cervicis m
4: Longissimus cervicis and longissimus capitis m
5: Semispinalis capitis m
6: Longissimus thoracis m
7: Levator costae m

Fig. **98**. Semispinalis capitis muscle.

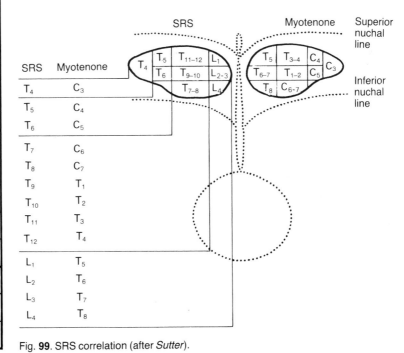

Fig. **99**. SRS correlation (after *Sutter*).

7.8.   Spinalis Muscle

The spinospinal system is made up of three muscles: the spinalis capitis, spinalis cervicis, and spinalis thoracis muscles. They interconnect the spinous processes and show great variability in their distribution. If present, the spinalis capitis muscle is fused anatomically with the semispinalis muscle.

We restrict the discussion to the spinalis thoracis muscle, which is the only one of some importance to manual therapeutic diagnosis.

7.8.1.   Spinalis Thoracis Muscle

Origin: spinous processes of T_{11}–$L_{2(3)}$, (Fig. **100**).

Insertion: tips of the spinous processes of (C_7) T_1–T_9 (Fig. **101**).

Course: The longest fasciculi run from L_3 to C_7 and T_1; the shortest, from T_{11} to T_8 or T_9. This arrangement results in the largest muscle profile in the lower thoracic region where the fibers can be palpated above the tips of the transverse processes (when myotendinosis is present) (Fig. **102**).

Innervation: dorsal rami of the thoracic nerves T_6–T_8.

Function: Bilateral contraction results in extension of the vertebral column, and unilateral contraction results in lateral flexion of the vertebral column.

Palpatory technique: The origin tendinosis of the spinalis thoracis muscle is palpated from a superior direction in order to reach the proximal pole of the spinous process. It must be differentiated from the adjoining origin tendinoses (such as that of the latissimus dorsi muscle in the lumbar region and serratus posterior inferior muscle in the upper thoracic and cervical region).

SRS correlation: The spinalis muscle is spondylogenically and reflexogenically correlated with the lumbar spine.

Remarks: As already noted, the spinalis cervicis and capitis muscles are nonuniform and, for all purposes, spondylogenically and reflexogenically insignificant.

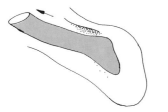

Fig. **100**. Origin of the spinalis muscle

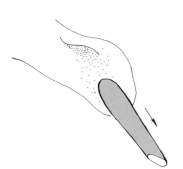

Fig. **101**. Insertion of the spinalis muscle

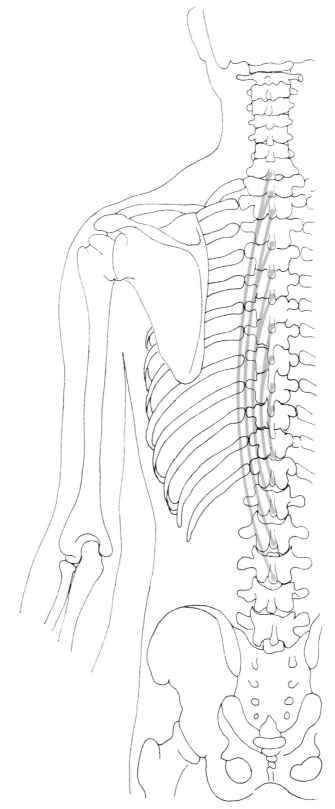

Fig. **102**. Schematic representation of the spinalis muscle.

7.9. Erector Spinae (Sacrospinales) Muscles-Organization

Origin (general): The longissimus and iliocostalis muscles are arranged anatomically in such a manner that their origins at the pelvis cannot be differentiated from one another. They share a common, remarkably broad origin, just like a two-headed muscle. Their origin extends from the spinous processes of all lumbar vertebrae via the median sacral crest, the posterior portion of the sacrum in the S_3–S_4 region, to the lateral sacral crest. It continues further to the medial and superior side of the iliac tuberosity, the short posterior sacroiliac ligaments and the anterior side of the posterior part of the inner lip of the crest of the ilium (Fig. **103**).

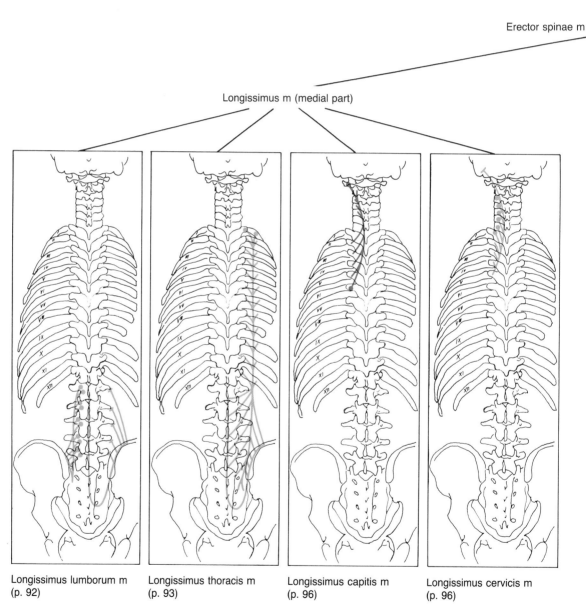

Erector spinae m

Longissimus m (medial part)

Longissimus lumborum m (p. 92)

Longissimus thoracis m (p. 93)

Longissimus capitis m (p. 96)

Longissimus cervicis m (p. 96)

Fig. **103**.

Iliocostalis m (lateral part)

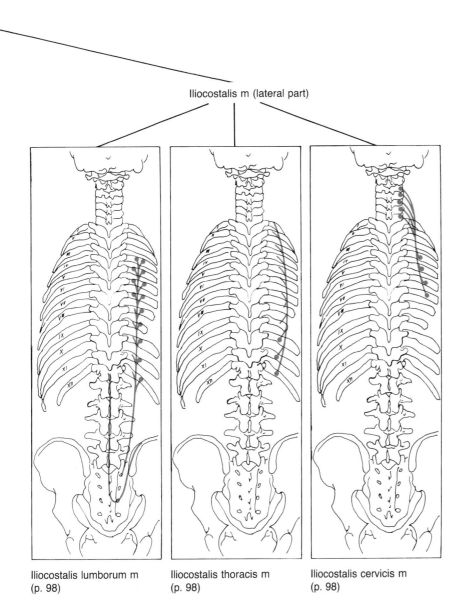

Iliocostalis lumborum m
(p. 98)

Iliocostalis thoracis m
(p. 98)

Iliocostalis cervicis m
(p. 98)

This division of the iliocostalis muscle into three portions is not complete, since it is normal
that smaller or larger portions of this muscle are continuous from one belly to another.

7.9.1. Longissimus Lumborum Muscle

Origin: The longissimus lumborum muscle arises from the broad sacrospinous ligament primarily at the superior and anterior portions of the iliac tuberosity (compare page 90).

Insertion: It inserts via two tendons at all lumbar vertebrae. A lateral row of broad insertions attaches to the entire inferior edge and the whole length of the posterior surface of the transverse processes of the lumbar vertebrae. The insertion at L_5 usually reaches only the iliolumbar ligament.

The medial row overlies the lateral row and converges toward the ligamentous fascia, above the mamillary and accessory processes. The dorsal ramus of the spinal nerves is located below this fascia.

Course and relations: The longissimus lumborum muscle lies deep in relation to the iliocostalis muscle and the longissimus thoracis muscle. By way of its origin at the iliac tuberosity, it connects to the interosseous sacroiliac ligaments.

Innervation: dorsal rami of the spinal nerve.

Function: Bilateral contraction results in extension of the column, and unilateral contraction results in lateral bending of the vertebral column to the side of the contracted muscle.

Palpatory technique: Except for very rare cases, it is almost impossible to palpate distinctly the origin tendinoses of the longissimus lumborum muscle. Thus, one must rely on the reporting of pain by the patient. The medial insertion tendinoses are determined from the inferior direction at the mamillary process. An often made mistake is the palpation from the posterior direction (or the origin of the transversospinal system).

The lateral portion is stronger than the medial and is palpated from the lateroinferior direction. One must attempt palpatory differentiation between this muscle and the lateral lumbar intertransverse muscles, whereby it should be noted that these two muscles can spondylogenically develop myotendinosis simultaneously.

SRS correlation: The insertions at the lateral and medial rows have different spondylogenic correlations: the lateral row of insertion is correlated with the first three sacral vertebrae, the medial one with the last cervical and the first four thoracic vertebrae (see table).

Remarks: The longissimus lumborum is a strong muscle. Myotendinosis of this muscle can cause a functionally abnormal position (segmental dysfunction) in a lumbar vertebra. In the case of the "functionally unstable pelvis" (according to SUTTER) a functionally abnormal position of the segments L_1, L_2, and L_3 can be caused by the lateral insertions that are correlated with S_1, S_2, and L_3. Due to the crossover of the SRS of L_1, L_2, and L_3, quite a complex clinical picture can arise in the skeleton as well as the extremities.

Spine	SRS Correlation			
C$_0$	L$_4$			
C$_1$	L$_5$			
C$_2$				
C$_3$				
C$_4$				
C$_5$	Medial line of insertions			
C$_6$				
C$_7$	L$_5$			
T$_1$	L$_4$			
T$_2$	L$_3$			
T$_3$	L$_2$			
T$_4$	L$_1$			
T$_5$				
T$_6$				
T$_7$				
T$_8$				
T$_9$				
T$_{10}$				
T$_{11}$				
T$_{12}$				
L$_1$				
L$_2$				
L$_3$				
L$_4$	Lateral line of insertions			
L$_5$				
S$_1$	L$_3$			
S$_2$	L$_1$			
S$_3$	L$_2$			

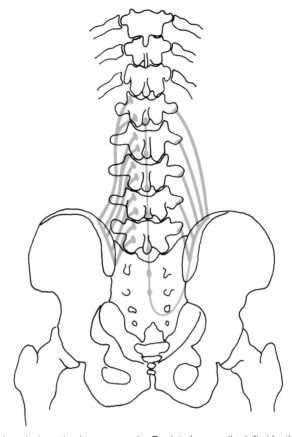

Fig. **104**. Longissimus lumborum muscle. Depicted are on the left side, the medial line of insertions of the longissimus lumborum muscle, and on the right side, the lateral line of insertions.

7.9.2. **Longissimus Thoracis Muscle**

Origin: See origin of the longissimus lumborum muscle.

Insertion: The insertions divide into two parts: the medial insertions (narrow) reach the tips of the transverse processes of the thoracic vertebrae (T_1–T_{12}) and the lateral insertions (broad) reach the ribs, in particular their inferior margin between the tubercle and costal angle. Some of its superior portions are strengthened through other muscle segments originating from the mamillary processes of L_1–L_2 (see sector V).

Course and relations: Muscle fibers originating at the iliac crest are destined for inferior insertions. The ones arriving from the lumbar spinous processes and the median sacral crest are directed toward the middle and upper thoracic spine (see sector division). The longissimus thoracis muscle lies lateral to the spinalis muscle and medial to the iliocostalis muscle, thus being on the midline over the thoracic transverse processes and lying laterally on the levatores costarum muscles and the ribs, reaching the line of the costal angle (Fig. **105**).

Innervation: dorsal rami of the spinal nerves.

Function: Bilateral contraction results in extension of the vertebral column, and unilateral contraction results in lateral bending of the vertebral column to the side of the contracted muscle.

Palpatory technique: Origins (compare sector division in Fig. **106**).

Sector I: The origin of sector I arises between the origins of the longissimus lumborum muscle on one side and the iliocostalis muscle on the other. The tendinoses at the iliac tuberosity and the intermediate line of the iliac crest are 4 to 8 mm broad. They are palpated posterosuperiorly in the direction of the iliac crest (differential diagnosis of the short sacroiliac ligaments).

Sector II: The tendinoses at the lateral sacral crest are also palpated posterosuperiorly (differential diagnosis of the long dorsal sacroiliac ligaments).

Sector IV: The origin is at the posterior aspect of the sacrum (S_3–S_4). These tendinoses are also 4 to 8 mm broad and must be distinguished from the sacral zones of irritation (ventralization testing). The palpatory direction is posterosuperior, according to the muscle fiber direction.

Sectors III and V: The origins of these two sectors are located at the spinous processes of L_1–L_3 (at the median sacral crest). The palpatory direction is in accordance with the muscle fiber direction when performed at the correct palpatory level and with the proper pressure. At L_1 and L_2 the superior reinforcement (see before) of the mamillary processes must be considered. Palpatory technique is modified accordingly.

Insertion: the same for all sectors: slight lateroinferiorly from posterior in the direction of the inferior lateral margin of the transverse process.

It is important to know that the insertion tendinosis of the longissimus thoracis muscle is almost always accompanied by the irritational zone of the corresponding thoracic vertebra (result of myotendinosis).

At the ribs, the insertions are palpated inferiorly, that is, between the tubercle and the costal angle at the inferior margin of the rib (comparison with the adjoining ribs is very important).

It is highly unlikely that the SRS correlation of these lateral lines of insertion is identical to that of the medial insertions. Since they have not been definitely categorized, they will not be treated here. The muscle overlying the hard surface of the ribs and the spinous processes can easily be palpated perpendicular to the fiber direction. This allows for the differential diagnosis of the adjoining muscle layers.

SRS-correlation: See the sector diagrams (Fig. **106**) and the table.

Remarks: The longissimus thoracis muscle is one of the most important muscles for the SRS. It responds quite rapidly to a functional disturbance, and myotendinosis usually results. It should not be difficult for persons with little palpatory experience to detect the myotendinosis of the longissimus thoracis muscle and to categorize it correctly.

Spine	SRS Correlation				
C₀					
C₁					
C₂					
C₃					
C₄					
C₅					
C₆					
C₇					
T₁					
T₂					
T₃					
T₄		Sector V			
T₅	T₁	L₁			
T₆	T₂	L₂			
T₇	T₃	L₁			
T₈	T₄	L₂	Sector II		
T₉			T₅	S₄	
T₁₀			T₆	S₄	
T₁₁			T₇	S₃	
T₁₂			T₈	S₃	
L₁	Sector III	L₂	L₃	Sector I	T₈
L₂	T₆		L₄		T₉
L₃	T₇	L₅	S₁		T₁₀
L₄	T₈	S₂	S₃		T₁₁
L₅	T₉		S₄		T₁₂
S₁	Sector IV	T₅	T₆		
S₂		T₉	T₁₀		
S₃		T₇	T₈		

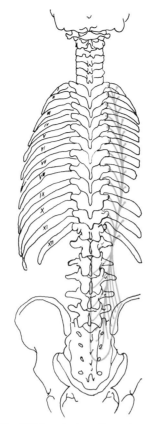

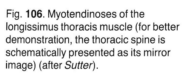

Fig. **105**. Longissimus thoracis muscle (schematic representation).

Fig. **106**. Myotendinoses of the longissimus thoracis muscle (for better demonstration, the thoracic spine is schematically presented as its mirror image) (after *Sutter*).

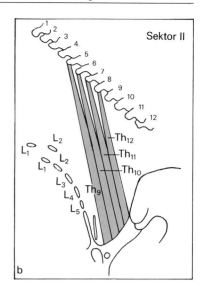

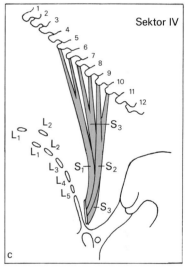

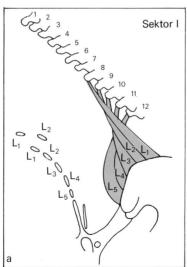

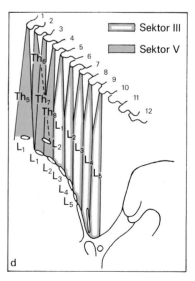

7.9.3. Longissimus Cervicis Muscle

Origin: the transverse processes of $T_{(1)2}$–T_6, close to the center of the superior surface of the tip. The muscle can reach T_8 in some cases.

Insertion: the posterior surface and root of the transverse processes (posterior tubercles) of $C_{(1)2}$–$C_{5(6-7)}$. It inserts practically together with the iliocostalis cervicis muscle, the splenius cervicis muscle, the levator scapulae muscle, the posterior scalene muscle, and the longissimus capitis muscle (Fig. **107**).

Course and relations: This is a flat, quite weak muscle with its main surface in the sagittal direction. At the T_4–T_5 level, it is often connected to the belly of the longissimus thoracis muscle via a tendon. In its lower half, it runs medially to the longissimus thoracis muscle. The muscle belly in the lower cervical region runs deeply and laterally to the longissimus capitis muscle, which in turn is lateral to the semispinalis capitis muscle. The muscle fiber direction is almost perfectly longitudinal. The longissimus group and the semispinalis capitis muscle have their own muscular fascia and can therefore be easily distinguished from each other by palpation (Fig. **108**).

Innervation: dorsal rami of the spinal nerve, the cervical nerves, and the thoracic nerves C_3–C_2.

Function: Unilateral contraction results in lateral bending of the cervical spine to the side of the contracted muscle, and bilateral contraction results in extension of the cervical spine.

Palpatory technique: The muscle belly is, as already described, easily palpable in the region of the lower cervical spine (perpendicular to the fiber direction).

The origins are palpated at the tip of the thoracic transverse processes from superior to inferior. It is very difficult to differentiate these origins from the semispinalis capitis and cervicis muscles (differential diagnosis at the insertion). The insertions at the posterior tubercle of the costal transverse processes are palpated from inferiorly to superiorly.

SRS correlation: Each origin to insertion unit represents one myotenone (that is, always the most superior insertion together with the most superior origin.)

The spondylogenic correlation of the individual myotenones can be seen in the table.

7.9.4. Longissimus Capitis Muscle

Origin: the transverse processes of $C_{(3-4)5}$–C_7 to T_1–$T_{3(5)}$. It arises at the cervical spine medial to the insertions and at the thoracic spine medial to the origins of the longissimus cervicis muscle.

Insertion: the posterior margin of the mastoid process to its tip with a length of 1.5 cm (Fig. **109**).

Course and relations: The longissimus capitis muscle is a slender muscle oriented in the sagittal plane. The longitudinal muscle bundles are arranged in such a manner that the bundles originating most inferiorly lie at the anterior edge of the muscle belly. In the deep layer of the lower cervical region, the muscle can easily be palpated between the semispinalis capitis and the longissimus cervicis muscle. It is covered at its insertion by the splenius capitis muscle and the sternocleidomastoid muscle (Fig. **110**).

Innervation: dorsal rami of the cervical nerves C_1–C_3, possibly C_4.

Function: Unilateral contraction results in lateral bending and rotation of the head to the side of the contracted muscle, and bilateral contraction results in extension of the head.

Palpatory technique: The muscle belly can easily be palpated perpendicularly to the fiber direction in the deep layers of the lower cervical region between the semispinalis capitis muscle and the longissimus muscle (see Figs. **53** and **55** of the cervical spine and thoracic spine cross-sections).

The insertion at the mastoid is palpated from posterioinferior to superior under the splenius capitis muscle and the sternocleidomastoid muscle from which it must be differentiated. The origins are palpated from superior to inferior in the direction of the root of the corresponding transverse processes.

SRS correlation: For this muscle as well, the muscular unit arising from one vertebra represents one myotenone. Its spondylogenic correlation can be seen in the table.

Differentiation of the individual myotendinoses at the insertion at the mastoid is impossible due to the concentration of ten myotenones in this small area. One can only palpate a painful insertion. A differential diagnosis is established with the aid of the origin tendinoses and the correlating zones of irritation.

Spine	SRS Correlation		
C_0			
C_1			
C_2			
C_3			
C_4			
C_5			
C_6	Longissimus cervicis m		Longissimus capitis m
C_7	C_1	T_2	C_3
T_1	C_2	T_3	C_4
T_2	C_3	T_4	C_5
T_3	C_4	T_5	C_6
T_4	C_5	T_6	C_7
T_5	(C_6)	(T_7)	T_1
T_6	(C_7)	(T_8)	T_2
T_7			T_3
T_8			T_4
T_9			T_5
T_{10}			
T_{11}			
T_{12}			
L_1			
L_2			
L_3			
L_4			
L_5			
S_1			
S_2			
S_3			

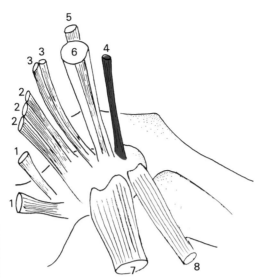

Fig. 107. Muscle attachments at the tip of the thoracic transverse process.

1: Rotatores muscles
2: Multifidus m
3: Semispinalis cervicis m
4: Longissimus cervicis m
5: Longissimus capitis m
6: Semispinalis capitis m
7: Longissimus thoracis m
8: Levator costae m.

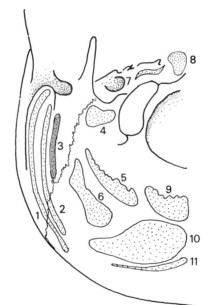

Fig. 109. Muscle attachments at the occiput.

1: Sternocleidomastoid m
2: Splenius capitis m
3: Longissimus capitis m
4: Rectus capitis lateralis m
5: Rectus capitis posterior major m
6: Obliquus capitis superior m
7: Rectus capitis anterior m
8: Longus capitis m
9: Rectus capitis posterior minor m
10: Semispinalis capitis m
11: Trapezius m

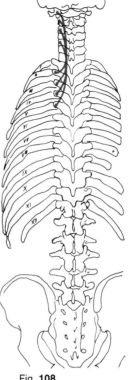

Fig. 108.
Longissimus cervicis m

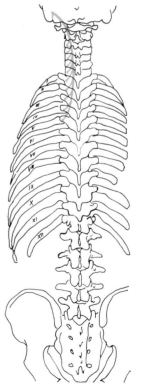

Fig. 110.
Longissimus capitis muscle

7.9.5. Iliocostalis Lumborum Muscle

Origin: the broad and thick sacrospinous ligament (see page 90), and the anterolateral surface of the iliac tuberosity.

Insertion: at the costal angle of ribs XII to IV (Fig. **111** a).

7.9.6. Iliocostalis Thoracis Muscle

Origin: medially at the costal angle of ribs XII to VII (Fig. **111** b).

Insertion: laterally at the costal angle of ribs VII to I (Fig. **111** b).

7.9.7. Iliocostalis Cervicis Muscle

Origin: directly medial to the costal angle of ribs VII to III (IV) (Fig. **111** c).

Insertion: at the posterior tubercles of the transverse processes of $C_{3(4)}$–C_6 (refer to the insertion of the longissimus cervicis muscle) (Fig. **111** c).

Course and relations: The iliocostalis muscle shows a tilelike architecture. The iliocostalis lumborum muscle ascends from inferior, traverses the posterior surfaces of the ribs going superiorly, and runs lateral to the longissimus thoracis muscle. In the neck region, the iliocostalis cervicis muscle lies also lateral to the longissimus cervicis and capitis muscle and medial to the posterior and medial scalene muscles as well as the levator scapulae muscle. Its main plane is in the sagittal direction. The iliocos-

talis cervicis muscle can be isolated anatomically but must be seen as the direct continuation of the iliocostalis lumborum muscle (Fig. **111** a–c).

Innervation: dorsal rami of the spinal nerves.

Function: Bilateral contraction results in extension of the vertebral column, and unilateral contraction results in lateral bending of the vertebral column to the side of the contracted muscle.

Palpatory technique: At its origin, the iliocostalis lumborum muscle cannot be distinguished from the tendon of the longissimus dorsi muscle. In its course we find the iliocostalis muscle to be lateral to the longissimus dorsi muscle. Inferiorly, we can palpate the insertion tendinoses at the inferior edge and the posterior surface of the costal angle. To avoid the contact with the levator costae muscle, the direction must be perfectly inferior.

The iliocostalis cervicis muscle can also be palpated easily. Its origins are palpated from medial-superior to lateral-inferior in the direction of costal angles. The insertions are palpated from inferior to superior at the posterior tubercles of the cervical transverse processes. During this maneuver, one has to differentiate between other muscles inserting at this location (longissimus cervicis muscle, levator scapulae muscle of C_3–C_4, scalene medial and posterior muscles, and the medial portion of the posterior cervical intertransverse muscles).

SRS correlation: The spondylogenic correlation of the iliocostalis muscle is still undetermined. Indications exist that the iliocostalis cervicis muscle is correlated with the myotenone L_5.

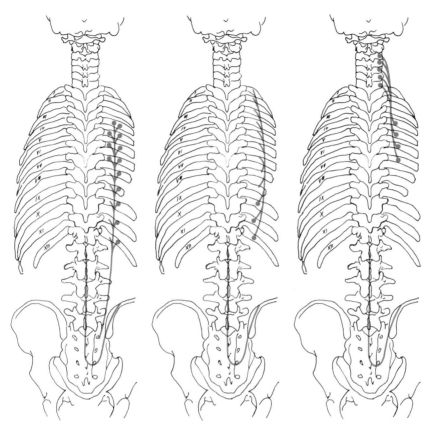

Fig. **111.**   (**a**) Iliocostalis lumborum m;   (**b**) Iliocostalis thoracis m;   (**c**) Iliocostalis cervicis m.

7.10. Splenius Muscle

This is a flat muscle that typically divides at its insertion into the splenius capitis and splenius cervicis muscles.

7.10.1. Splenius Capitis Muscle

Origin: the nuchal ligament: inferior to and including C_3. Further, from the spinous processes of C_7 and T_1–T_3 and the supraspinous ligament (Fig. **113**).

Insertion: at the lateral surface of the mastoid process, including its tip. This insertion forms a posterior arch reaching the lateral half of the superior nuchal line (Fig. **112**).

7.10.2. Splenius Cervicis Muscle

Origin: The spinous processes and the supraspinous ligaments of T_3–$T_{5(6)}$. The length of the tendons increases inferiorly. The parallel muscle bundles form a long, slender belly that is more vertical than that of the splenius capitis muscle and swings around the neck superolaterally.

Insertion: via three tendons of disproportionate strength. The strongest fascicle inserts in the posteroinferior portion of the tip of the transverse process of the atlas, the second strongest, at the tip of the transverse process of the axis, and the third, at the posterior surface of the transverse process of C_3 (Fig. **113**).

Course and relation: A broad section of the inferior and medial portions of the splenius muscle is covered by the trapezius muscle, the rhomboid muscle, and the serratus posterior superior muscle. The sternocleidomastoid and the levator scapulae muscles cover the splenius muscle superiorly and laterally. The splenius muscle overlies the semispinalis capitis muscle (see Fig. **53**, the cervical spine cross-section). Many parts of the inserting tendons of the splenius cervicis muscles are fused with the tendons of the levator scapulae muscle and the longissimus cervicis muscle. The free medial border of the splenius capitis muscle forms together with the nuchal ligament and the medial end of the superior nuchal line, a triangular space through which the occipital vessels and the greater occipital nerve emerge.

Innervation: dorsal rami of the cervical nerves C_1–C_5.

Function: Bilateral contraction results in extension of the head and the cervical spine, and unilateral contraction results in lateral bending and rotation of the head to the side of the contracted muscle.

Palpatory technique: Due to the flat nature of these muscles, palpation is difficult. The spinous process of C_3 is palpated first superolaterally. One continues inferiorly through C_4–C_5 to T_5–T_6, staying at the surface. The palpatory direction is almost vertical in the inferior segments. The inserting portion of the splenius capitis muscle is palpated inferiorly at the lateral surface of the mastoid process and is then followed in an arch to the superior nuchal line. The strongest insertion tendon of the splenius cervicis muscle is palpated posteroinferior in direction of the tip of the transverse process of the atlas. The inserting tendons leading to C_2 and C_3 are substantially weaker and are palpated from a posteroinferior direction as well.

SRS correlation: Both the splenius capitis and the splenius cervicis muscles are correlated with the vertebra of C_7 as one single myotenone.

Remarks: The splenius cervicis muscle traverses the zone of irritation of C_7, which can often lead to confusion with myotendinotic changes of the splenius capitis muscle. One can avoid this situation, however, by flexing the head laterally (relaxation and displacement of the splenius cervicis muscle).

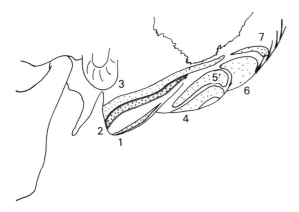

Fig. **112**. Muscle attachments at the mastoid process and the occiput.

1: Longissimus capitis m
2: Splenius capitis m
3: Sternocleidomastoid m
4: Rectus capitis posterior major m
5: Obliquus capitis superior m
6: Semispinalis capitis m
7: Trapezius m

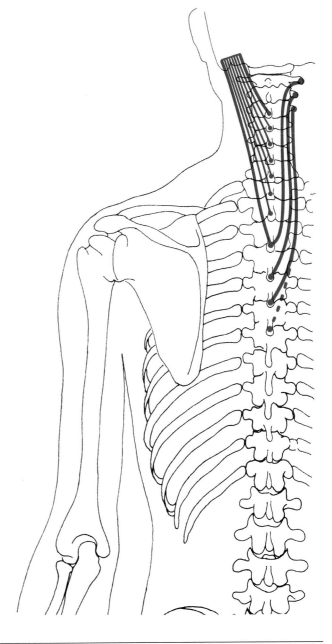

Fig. **113**. Splenius capitis muscle on the left, splenius cervicis muscle on the right.

7.11. Levatores Costarum (Longi and Breves) Muscles

The levatores costarum muscles are short and strong and are only found alongside the thoracic spine. They owe their name to their action of lifting the ribs. There are 12 pairs of short levatores costarum muscles, and only four pairs of the long levatores costarum muscles are developed, those for the four most inferior ribs. Here, they are discussed collectively, even though their SRS correlation is different.

Origin: the posterior tubercle of the transverse processes of C_7 the inferior margin of the thick tip of the transverse processes of T_I–T_{II}, sometimes including its base.

Insertion: The levatores costarum muscles insert at the superoposterior surface of the ribs, that is, between the tubercle and the costal angle. The short levatores costarum muscles insert into the outer surface of the rib immediately below their respective origins. In contrast, the long levatores costarum muscles skip the rib immediately inferior and therefore insert two ribs below their respective origin.

Course and relations: The levatores costarum muscles are found at the same level as the short deep muscles of the back (such as the intertransverse muscles and rotatores muscles). Thus, they lie under the muscle masses of the long and superficial back musculature (see Fig. **55** the cross-section of the thoracic spine).

The direction of the muscles from their origin to their insertion at the ribs is lateroinferior (Fig. **114**).

Innervation: the intercostal nerves, T_1–T_{11}.

Function: even though the levatores costarum muscles insert at the ribs, they belong functionally to the deep back muscles, rather than to the intercostales muscles. Bilateral contraction results in extension of the thoracic spine, and unilateral contraction results in rotation of the vertebral column to the opposite side and lateral bending of the vertebral column to the side of the contracted muscle.

Palpatory technique: The close relationship to both the longissimus thoracis muscle at the origin and the iliocostalis thoracis muscle at the insertion, which cover these small muscles, for the most part, requires a precise palpatory direction. First the thumb locates the myotendinosis perpendicular to the direction of the fibers and then follows the muscle in order to determine the tendinoses.

SRS correlation: See table. These muscles, which have a very small diameter, are often responsible for certain vertebral and rib lesions, that is, the so-called blocked rib. This situation must be diagnosed via provocative testing. The pattern resulting from the zone of irritation dictates the adequate therapy both for the vertebra and the rib.

Spine	SRS Correlation			
C_0				
C_1				
C_2				
C_3				
C_4				
C_5				
C_6				
C_7	Breves			
T_1	C_0			
T_2	C_1			
T_3	C_2			
T_4	C_3			
T_5	C_4			
T_6	C_5	Longi		
T_7	C_6	C_5		
T_8	C_7	C_4		
T_9	T_1	C_3		
T_{10}	T_2	C_2		
T_{11}	T_3			
T_{12}				
L_1				
L_2				
L_3				
L_4				
L_5				
S_1				
S_2				
S_3				

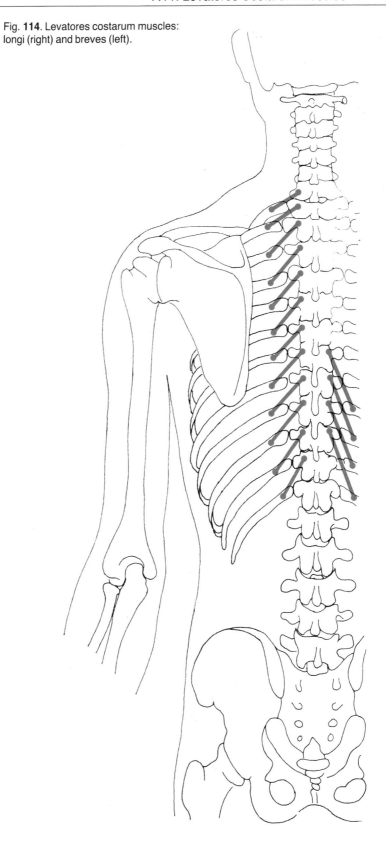

Fig. **114**. Levatores costarum muscles: longi (right) and breves (left).

7.12. Scalene Muscles

7.12.1. Anterior Scalene Muscle

Origin: This muscle arises as four tendons from the anterior tubercles of the transverse processes of C_3–C_6. The strongest, fleshy tendinous slip arises from the anterior tubercle (tuberculum caroticum) of C_6.

Insertion: tubercle of the anterior scalene muscle at the upper first rib (Figs. **115, 116**).

7.12.2. Middle Scalene Muscle

Origin: posterior margin of the groove for the spinal nerve and the posterior tubercles of the transverse processes of C_3–C_7 (Fig. **115**).

Insertion: This muscle inserts along the entire width of the first rib, behind the subclavian roof, with tendinous insertion in the fascia of the first intercostal space (outer thoracic surface), and sometimes at the superior edge of the second rib (Fig. **116**).

7.12.3. Posterior Scalene Muscle

Origin: the posterior tubercles of the transverse processes of C_6 and C_7.

Insertion: This muscle inserts as a thin aponeurosis at the outer surface of the second rib (next to the tuberosity for the serratus anterior muscle) (Fig. 117).

Course and relations: The spatial arrangement of the scalene muscles can be deduced from their name. The anterior scalene muscle lies lateral to the inferior portion of the longus colli muscle. The middle scalene muscle lies posterolaterally to the scalene anterior muscle, and the posterior scalene muscle lies posteriorly to the middle scalene muscle. The fiber direction of the the three muscles is lateroinferior.

In contrast to the anterior and middle scalene muscles, the posterior scalene muscle traverses the first rib and inserts at the second rib.

When palpating, one has to be aware of the close relationship of the scalene muscles with the subclavian artery and the brachial plexus.

Innervation: the ventral rami of the cervical spinal nerves (C_3–C_8).

Function: Bilateral contraction results in flexion of the cervical spine, and unilateral contraction results in bending to the side of the contracted muscle, with opposite rotation of the cervical spine. When the cervical spine is fixed, the muscle raises the second rib.

Palpatory technique: The origin tendinoses at the anterior and posterior tubercles are palpated anteroinferiorly. The origins can easily be reached with the finger used for palpation. The insertions at the first rib (anterior and middle scalene muscles) are palpated superiorly, behind the clavicles in the thoracic inlet. It should be noted that the patient finds this palpatory procedure extremely uncomfortable which is primarily attributable to the brachial plexus. The insertion of the posterior scalene muscle is palpated at the second rib, from posterosuperior, about two finger widths lateral to the end of the transverse process of T_2. Since one has to palpate through the trapezius muscle, the palpatory findings are not easily elicited.

SRS correlation: The myotendinosis of the anterior scalene muscle may cause a "functionally abnormal position" (segmental dysfunction) at the cervical spine in the anterior direction, similar to the myotendinosis of the longus colli muscle (the more anterior the segmental dysfunction, the stronger the zone of irritation). As can be seen from the table, the scalene muscle myotenones are correlated with the central portion of the thoracic spine.

Remarks: The so-called elevated rib is normally the result of myotendinosis in one part of the scalene muscles.

Spine	SRS Correlation			
C$_0$				
C$_1$				
C$_2$				
C$_3$				
C$_4$				
C$_5$				
C$_6$				
C$_7$				
T$_1$		medius		
T$_2$		C$_3$		
T$_3$		C$_4$		
T$_4$	C$_6$	C$_5$		
T$_5$	C$_5$	C$_6$		
T$_6$	C$_4$	C$_7$	posterior	
T$_7$	C$_3$		C$_6$	
T$_8$			C$_7$	
T$_9$				
T$_{10}$				
T$_{11}$				
T$_{12}$				
L$_1$				
L$_2$				
L$_3$				
L$_4$				
L$_5$				
S$_1$				
S$_2$				
S$_3$				

(anterior — label spanning the first sub-column at T3/T4)

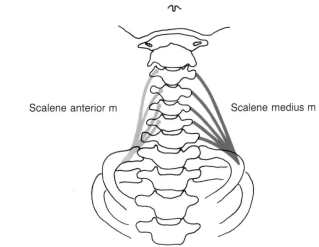

Scalene anterior m   Scalene medius m

Fig. **115**. Scalene muscles.

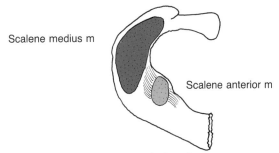

Scalene medius m

Scalene anterior m

Fig. **116**. Muscle attachments at the first rib.

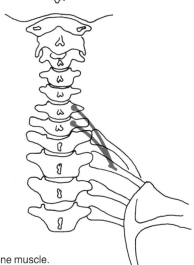

Fig. **117**. Posterior scalene muscle.

7.13. Muscles of the Serratus Group

7.13.1. Anterior Serratus Muscle

Origin: The anterior serratus muscle arises by nine, sometimes ten, strong fasciculi from the convex portion of the body ribs I to IX (X). The four most inferior fasciculi slide below the insertions of the external abdominal oblique muscle (Fig. **118**).

Insertion: The muscle inserts at the costal surface of the medial margin of the scapula, between the superior and inferior angle. Fibers arising from the first and second rib insert at the superior angle, and those arising from the third and fourth rib insert at the center of the medial margin. The remaining muscle fibers, the strongest, arise from ribs V to X in a fan-shaped pattern. They insert at the inferior angle of the scapula (Fig. **119**).

Innervation: long thoracic nerve from C_5–C_7.

Function: The anterior serratus muscle draws the scapula forward, away from the vertebral column; primarily, the inferior portions rotate the scapula so that the glenoid cavity points in a superior direction (abduction of the arm beyond the horizontal).

Palpation: Starting with the fourth rib and below the origin fasciculi are easily palpated, even without pathological muscle changes. At the lateral thoracic wall, the fasciculi are palpated posteriorly. In order to reach the insertion, the scapula must be elevated at the inferior angle. The finger follows along the costal surface of the medial margin as far as possible.

SRS correlation: See table. Involved in the spondylogenic event are most often the myotenones arising from the sixth and seventh ribs; these myotenones are also responsible for the corresponding abnormal position of the ribs.

Spine	SRS Correlation			
C_0				
C_1				
C_2				
C_3				
C_4				
C_5		Rib		
C_6		(X.)		
C_7		(IX.)		
T_1		VIII.		
T_2		VII.		
T_3		VI.		
T_4		V.		
T_5		IV.		
T_6		III.		
T_7		II.		
T_8		I.		
T_9				
T_{10}				
T_{11}				
T_{12}				
L_1				
L_2				
L_3				
L_4				
L_5				
S_1				
S_2				
S_3				

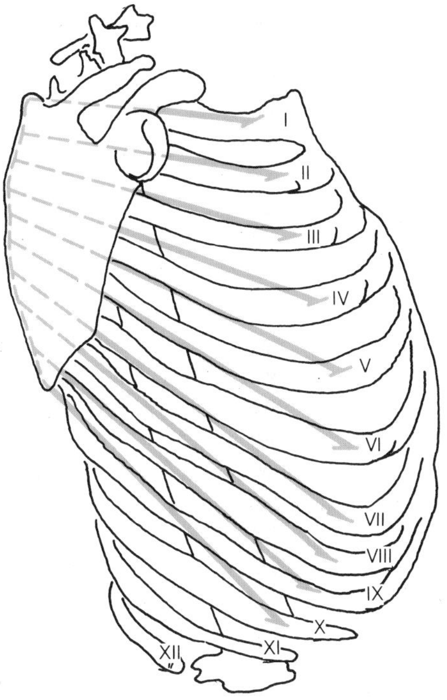

Fig. **118**. Anterior serratus muscle.

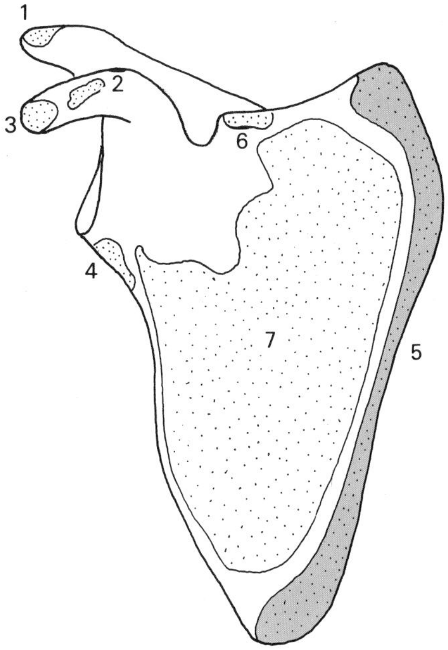

1: Deltoid m
2: Pectoralis minor m
3: Coracobrachialis m
Biceps brachii m (short head)
4: Triceps brachii m (long head)
5: Serratus anterior m
6: Omohyoid m
7: Subscapularis m

Fig. **119**. Muscle attachments at the anterior side of the scapula.

7.13.2. Serratus Posterior Superior Muscle

Origin: The muscle arises from the nuchal ligament close to the spinous process of C_6 and from the tips of the spinous processes of C_7, T_1, T_2.

Insertion: The muscle inserts by four fasciculi at ribs II to V, lateral to the costal angles.

Course and relations: This deep muscle runs from the spinous processes to the ribs at an angle of about $30°$ and is primarily covered by the rhomboid and the trapezius muscles (Fig. **120**).

Innervation: intercostal nerves of T_1–T_4.

Function: elevation of the ribs.

Palpation: This deep muscle can be palpated at the spinous processes only from an inferolateral direction, which in turn is only possible when the insertion tendinoses are localized and when differentiated from the spondylogenic correlation with the rhomboid muscle.

7.13.3. Seratus Posterior Inferior Muscle

Origin: the spinous processes and the supraspinous ligament T_{11}–$L_{2(3)}$. The tendon of the origin of the serratus posterior inferior muscle is practically identical with the superficial layer of the thoracolumbar fascia and the lumbar origin aponeurosis of the latissimus dorsi muscle (Fig. **120**).

Insertion: The serratus posterior inferior muscle inserts by four fasciculi at the inferior margin of ribs IX to XII between the origins of the latissimus dorsi muscle and the iliocostalis muscle. The most lateral fibers travel to the ninth rib almost horizontally.

Course and relations: This muscle, which shows an almost perfectly horizontal course, is only covered by the latissimus dorsi muscle. The tendon and muscle junction is located at the lateral edge of the iliocostalis muscle, where one can often find a painful myotendinosis.

Innervation: intercostal nerves T_9–T_{12}.

Function: fixation of the four most inferior ribs (resistance to diaphragm contraction), therefore considered to support inspiration.

Palpation: Even though the serratus posterior inferior muscle is completely covered by the latissimus dorsi muscle, myotendinosis can be palpated very well.

The palpatory direction is perpendicular to the fiber direction, from inferior to superior. The insertion tendinoses are located at the ribs about four finger widths lateral to the spinous processes.

SRS correlation: Both the serratus posterior superior muscle and the serratus posterior inferior muscle each represent one individual myotenone. Their correlation can be seen from the table.

Spine	SRS Correlation			
C_0				
C_1				
C_2				
C_3				
C_4				
C_5				
C_6				
C_7				
T_1	C_6	C_7	T_1	T_2
T_2				
T_3				
T_4				
T_5				
T_6				
T_7				
T_8				
T_9				
T_{10}				
T_{11}				
T_{12}				
L_1	T_{11}	L_1	L_2	L_3
L_2				
L_3				
L_4				
L_5				
S_1				
S_2				
S_3				

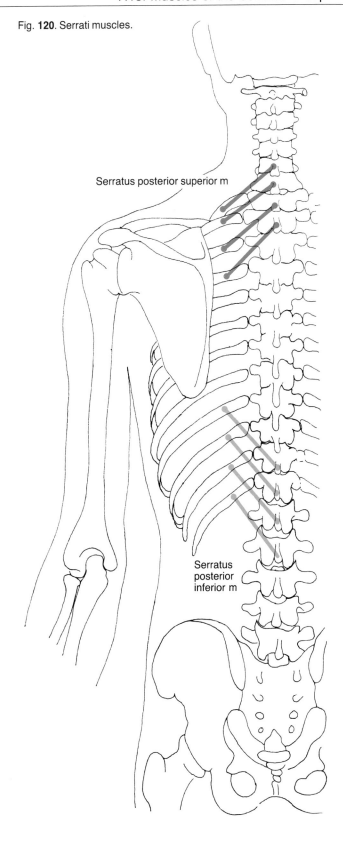

Fig. **120**. Serrati muscles.

Serratus posterior superior m

Serratus posterior inferior m

7.14. Levator Scapulae Muscle

Origin: The levator scapulae muscle arises by four fasciculi from the transverse processes of the first four cervical vertebrae. The first, the strongest, origin tendon reaches around the transverse process of the atlas lateroanteriorly. The origin tendons from C_2 to C_4 arise from the posterior tubercles. The first two fasciculi are completely fused with the tendons of the splenius cervicis muscle, and the last two are commonly fused with the longissimus cervicis muscle (Fig. **121**).

Insertion: The muscle inserts at the medial border of the scapula between the superior angle and the base of the scapular spine. The muscle bundles from C_1 insert immediately below the superior angle of the scapula. The insertions of the muscle fibers originating from C_2 to C_4 reach the base of the spine of the scapula at an extremely sharp angle (Fig. **122**).

Course and relations: The levator scapulae muscle is located laterally at the neck, between the anterior and posterior muscle mass and from C_5–C_6 on is covered by fibers of the trapezius muscles.

Innervation: the cervical plexus and the nerve of the rhomboids (n. dorsalis scapulae C_3–C_5).

Function: elevation of the scapula. When the scapula is fixed, it bends the neck laterally to the side of the contracted muscle.

Palpatory technique: Palpation cannot differentiate between the origins of this muscle and other muscles originating in close proximity (see Fig. **53** for a diagram of the cervical spine). The insertion tendinosis at the medial border of the scapula, however, can clearly be identified. Due to the steeply angled insertion, the palpatory direction is from the superior direction.

SRS correlation: See table.

Remarks: When myotendinotic changes affect both the levator scapulae muscle and the descending part of the trapezius muscle, an extremely painful "cross-myosis" at the T_1 level often develops about three finger widths from the spinous process and thus complicates the correct manipulation of C_3 and C_4.

7.15. Rhomboid Major and Minor Muscles

Origin: The rhomboid minor muscle arises via a short aponeurosis from the nuchal ligament at the C_6 level and from the spinous process of C_7; the rhomboid major arises from the spinous processes of T_1–T_4, rudimentarily from T_5 (Fig. **123**).

Insertion: the medial border of the scapula: the rhomboid minor muscle inserts at the level of the spine of the scapula; the rhomboid major muscle inserts distally to the base of the spine of the scapula (Fig. **124**).

Innervation: nerve of the rhomboids (n. dorsalis scapulae C_4, C_5).

Function: elevation and drawing of the scapula medially.

Palpatory technique: The close relationship to the trapezius muscle (horizontal portion) requires that the finger during palpation presses deeply from the lateroinferior direction; a definitive differentiation is possible at the medial border of the scapula due to the insertion tendinoses, which are approached mediosuperiorly.

SRS correlation: See table.

Remarks: Both rhomboid muscles often participate in the spondylogenic event; clinically, patients indicate pain between the shoulder blades.

Spine	SRS Correlation			
C_0				
C_1				
C_2		Rhomboid minor/major muscle		
C_3				
C_4			C_7	
C_5				T_1
C_6				T_2
C_7				T_3
T_1	Levator scapulae m			T_4
T_2	C_1			T_5
T_3	C_2			
T_4	C_3			
T_5	C_4			
T_6				
T_7				
T_8				
T_9				
T_{10}				
T_{11}				
T_{12}				
L_1				
L_2				
L_3				
L_4				
L_5				
S_1				
S_2				
S_3				

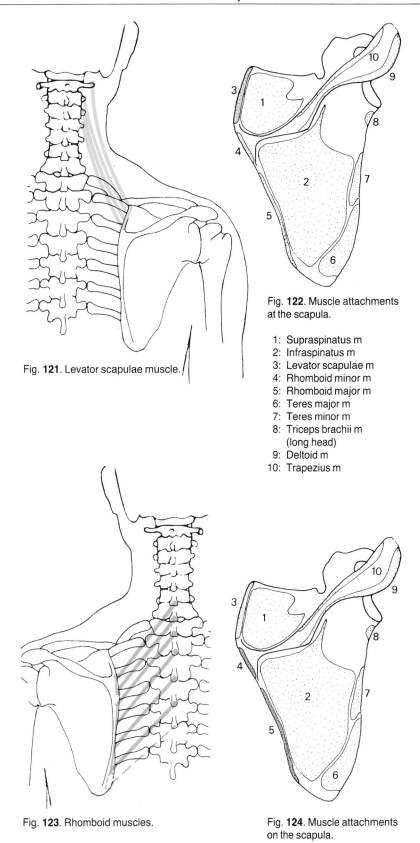

Fig. **121**. Levator scapulae muscle.

Fig. **122**. Muscle attachments at the scapula.

1: Supraspinatus m
2: Infraspinatus m
3: Levator scapulae m
4: Rhomboid minor m
5: Rhomboid major m
6: Teres major m
7: Teres minor m
8: Triceps brachii m (long head)
9: Deltoid m
10: Trapezius m

Fig. **123**. Rhomboid muscles.

Fig. **124**. Muscle attachments on the scapula.

7.16. Latissimus Dorsi Muscle

Origin:

1. Vertebral region: from the spinous processes and the supraspinous ligaments ($T_{(7)8}$–L_5, possibly from the median sacral crest (Fig. **125**).

2. Iliac region: from the external lip of the iliac crest, at the junction of the iliac tuberosity and the iliac crest; about four finger widths broad.

3. Costal region: as thin fasciculi from the outer surfaces of ribs X to XII; between the origins of the obliquus externus abdominis muscle and the insertions of the serratus posterior inferior muscle.

4. Thoracolumbar fascia

Insertion: the proximal end of the crest of the lesser tuberosity, connecting distally to the insertion of the subscapularis muscle. The proximal portion of the insertion belongs to the distal vertebral, iliac, and costal myotenones, the distal portion to the proximal vertebral myotenones, causing the latissimus dorsi muscle to be somewhat twisted (Fig. **126**).

Course and relations: The superior bundles run horizontally above the inferior angle of the scapula and the origin of the teres major muscle. In the axilla the muscle, which otherwise is flat, becomes considerably thick.

The lateral edge of the muscle descends from the axilla to the ilium quite vertically.

Innervation: thoracodorsal nerves C_6–C_8.

Function: adduction, extension, and medial rotation of the arm. The costal origins aid in inspiration.

Palpatory technique: The iliac crest, the latissimus dorsi muscle, and the external abdominal oblique muscle form the lumbar triangle (Petiti). Due to the flat origin aponeurosis, myotendinosis in the lumbar region is almost impossible to palpate. We gain better information about the muscle in the posterior axillary fold. When investigating the condition of the latissimus dorsi muscle, the approach is similar to the descending portion of the trapezius muscle. The myotendinosis is palpated perpendicular to the muscle fiber orientation in both directions: superiorly to the insertion at the crest of the lesser tuberosity and inferiorly. At the spinous processes, the origin of the latissimus dorsi, which is often painful, must be distinguished from the longissimus thoracis muscle, which lies below. The myotendinosis of this flat muscle can be palpated quite distinctly from rib to rib above their hard surface.

SRS correlation: The myotenones arising from the iliac crest are influenced spondylogenically by the segments of C_5 and C_6, whereas vertebral myotenones are influenced by the segments of C_7–T_5 (see table).

Remarks: The latissimus dorsi muscle is very often involved in the spondylogenic event. Patients indicate a rather fan-shaped, constant pain in the lumbar spine region.

Spine	SRS Correlation			
C₀				
C₁				
C₂		Crista		
C₃		Crista		
C₄		Crista		
C₅		C₂	C₃	
C₆		C₁		
C₇		L₅		
T₁		L₃	L₄	
T₂		L₁	L₂	
T₃		T₁₁	T₁₂	
T₄		T₉	T₁₀	
T₅		(T₇)	T₈	
T₆				
T₇				
T₈				
T₉				
T₁₀				
T₁₁				
T₁₂				
L₁				
L₂				
L₃				
L₄				
L₅				
S₁				
S₂				
S₃				

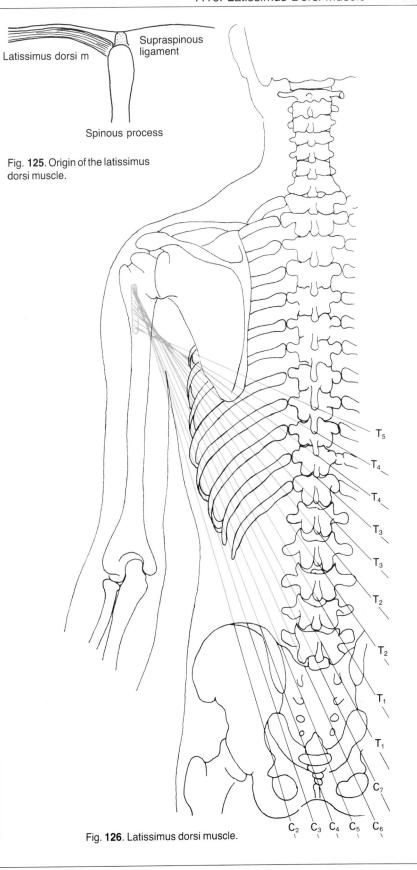

Latissimus dorsi m

Supraspinous ligament

Spinous process

Fig. **125**. Origin of the latissimus dorsi muscle.

Fig. **126**. Latissimus dorsi muscle.

7.17. Trapezius Muscle

Origin: The origin of the trapezius muscle extends between the occipital bone and the twelfth thoracic vertebra. It is useful to anatomically and spondylogenically divide this muscle into three sections: the descending, horizontal, and ascending portions (Fig. **127**).

Descending portion: the muscle arises from the superior nuchal line, 2 cm lateral to the external occipital protuberance; the nuchal ligament to the sixth cervical vertebra.

Horizontal portion: the spinous processes of C_7–T_3.

Ascending portion: the spinous processes of T_4–T_{12}.

Insertion: *Descending portion:* the superior surface of the spine of the scapula, the acromioclavicular joint, and the posterosuperior margin of the lateral third of the clavicle (Fig. **128**).

Horizontal portion: the superior surface of the spine of the scapula from the base to the acromioclavicular joint. At the spine of the scapula, this portion covers the insertion of the descending portion (important for palpation) (Fig. **128**).

Ascending portion: the inferior edge of the spine of the scapula, between the tuberosity and the lumbar triangle (Fig. **128**).

Course and relations: The muscle bundles arising from the occipital bone run sharply inferiorly, whereas the fibers continuing below course away from the ligamentum nuchae at quite a sharp angle. The fibers from the most inferior portion of the cervical spine approximate the transverse direction (Fig. **128**).

Innervation: the descending portion of the spinal accessory nerve and the rami of the cervical plexus C_2–C_4.

Function: *Descending portion:* elevation of the shoulder blade.

Horizontal portion: adduction of the scapula.

Ascending portion: pulling down of the scapula.

Palpatory technique: Since the trapezius muscle is located subcutaneously, palpating it serves as good training for the beginner. All anatomic structures can be exactly located and easily reached. To gain an overview whether myotendinotic changes are present, the muscle belly of the descending portion is grasped halfway between the shoulder and the neck between the thumb and index finger, upon which one moves up and down perpendicular in the direction of the muscle fibers. At the spinous processes, the spine of the scapula, and the clavicles, the tendinoses must be palpated in the direction of the incoming fibers (Fig. **128**). It should be noted that the descending and ascending portions are partially covered at the spine of the scapula by fibers of the horizontal portion.

SRS correlation: The trapezius muscle is extremely important for routine diagnosis of the SRS. Seldom is the trapezius muscle responsible for the abnormal position of individual vertebrae. In contrast, individual myotenones result in painful pathological changes (myotendinosis) when problems in the region of the thoracic and lumbar vertebra arise. When the muscle is palpated precisely, the spondylogenic pathology of the entire thoracic and lumbar spine can be deduced. The spondylogenic correlation of the myotenones is indicated in the table, for the descending portion in Figure **128a** (myotenones), for the horizontal and ascending portions in Figure **128b**.

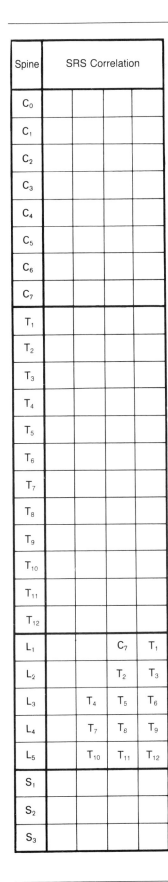

Spine	SRS Correlation			
C_0				
C_1				
C_2				
C_3				
C_4				
C_5				
C_6				
C_7				
T_1				
T_2				
T_3				
T_4				
T_5				
T_6				
T_7				
T_8				
T_9				
T_{10}				
T_{11}				
T_{12}				
L_1			C_7	T_1
L_2			T_2	T_3
L_3		T_4	T_5	T_6
L_4		T_7	T_8	T_9
L_5		T_{10}	T_{11}	T_{12}
S_1				
S_2				
S_3				

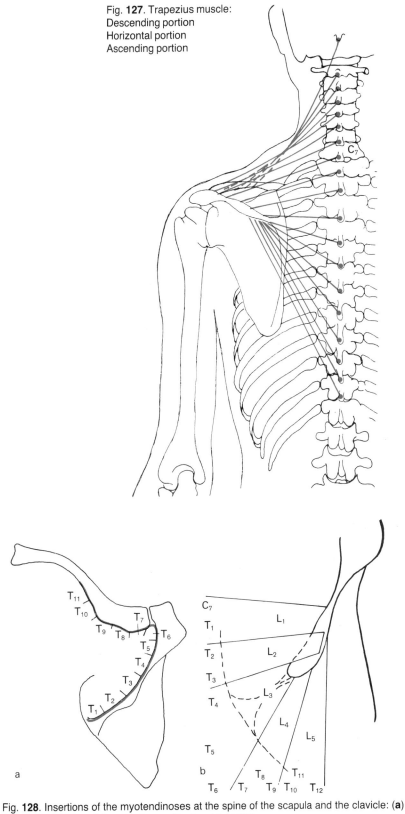

Fig. **127**. Trapezius muscle:
Descending portion
Horizontal portion
Ascending portion

Fig. **128**. Insertions of the myotendinoses at the spine of the scapula and the clavicle: (**a**) descending portion; (**b**) ascending and horizontal portion.

7.18. Quadratus Lumborum Muscle

Anatomically as well as spondylogenically, this muscle consists of superficial (posterior) and deep (anterior) layers.

Superficial (Posterior) Layer: (Fig. **129**).

Origin: The origin of this muscle spreads over the horizontal portion of the internal lip of the iliac crest (about 6 cm long; partially from the iliolumbar ligament).

Insertion: the anterior side of the tips of the costal processes L_1–L_4, some of the fibers radiate to the iliolumbar ligament (L_5). The most anterior fibers reach to the twelfth rib.

Palpatory technique: Due to its position, it cannot be palpated easily. Confusion, especially with the longissimus lumborum muscle, is possible. The palpating finger must reach around the iliac crest superiorly in a hooklike manner in order to reach the painful tendinoses. The insertions at the tips of the costal processes are palpated lateroinferiorly (L_4 can be palpated sometimes, whereas L_5 is practically never palpated).

Deep (Anterior) Layer: (Fig. **130**).

Origin: the inferior margin of the medial half of rib XII.

Insertion: The medial fibers insert at the anterior portion of the tips of the costal processes of L_1–L_5; the lateral fibers insert at the iliac crest, in about the same region as the superficial layer.

Course and relations: The posterior surface of the quadratus lumborum muscle lies over the deep portion of the thoracolumbar fascia of the aponeurosis of the transverse abdominis and the internal abdominal oblique muscles. The anterior portion borders on the kidneys and the colon. The psoas major muscle slides over the medial margin, and the quadratus lumborum muscle is laterally covered by the thick mass of the deep back muscles. In the inferior quarter it is covered by the pelvic portion of the latissimus dorsi muscle.

Innervation: the subcostal nerve and ventral ramus (n. lumbalis) T_{12} and L_1–L_3.

Function: Bilateral contraction results in extension of the lumbar spine, and unilateral contraction results in lateral bending of the vertebral column to the side of the contracted muscle. In addition, the muscle fixes the twelfth rib. It therefore facilitates diaphragm contraction.

Palpatory technique: The tendinoses at the twelfth rib, which often are painful, are palpated medioinferiorly, and the costal processes are palpated laterosuperiorly.

SRS correlation: See table and Figure **131**.

Spine	SRS Correlation			
C_0				
C_1				
C_2				
C_3				
C_4	posterior			
C_5	L_5			
C_6	L_4			
C_7	L_3			
T_1	L_2			
T_2	L_1			
T_3				
T_4				
T_5				
T_6				
T_7	anterior			
T_8	L_1			
T_9	L_2			
T_{10}	L_3			
T_{11}	L_4			
T_{12}	L_5			
L_1				
L_2				
L_3				
L_4				
L_5				
S_1				
S_2				
S_3				

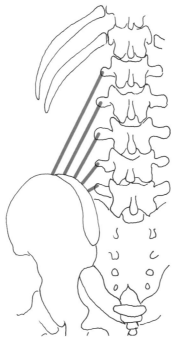

Fig. **129**. Quadratus lumborum muscle (superficial layer).

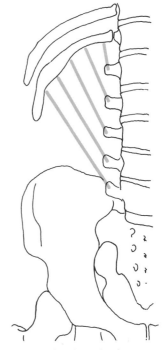

Fig. **130**. Quadratus lumborum muscle (deep layer).

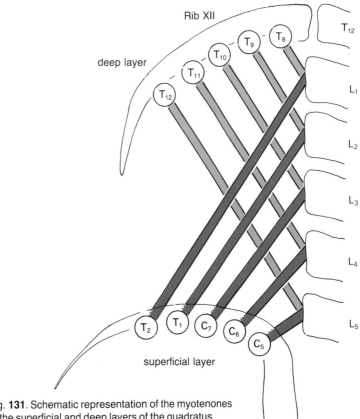

Fig. **131**. Schematic representation of the myotenones of the superficial and deep layers of the quadratus lumborum muscle (from posterior).

7.19. Psoas Major Muscle

Origin: It arises from the anteroinferior surfaces of the transverse processes L_1–L_5, not including the tips (where the quadratus lumborum muscle arises). The origin at L_5 covers the complete anterior surface. Furthermore, the psoas major muscle arises from the lateral and lateroanterior circumference of the intervertebral discs of T_{12}–L_5 and their respective vertebral bodies of L_1–L_4 (Fig. **132**).

Insertion: the anterior half of the lesser trochanter of the femur.

Course and relations: The muscle runs downward, alongside the lumbar spine (psoas shadow in x-rays) into the true pelvis and, below the inguinal ligament, through the lacuna musculorum (ilium) to the lesser trochanter. Upon exit from the lacuna musculorum, the muscle lies directly on the anterior side of the hip joint.

Innervation: rami of the lumbar plexus and the femoral nerve. The psoas major and minor muscles are segmentally innervated by L_1–L_3, sometimes by T_{12} and L_4.

Function: flexion of the thigh, possibly adduction and lateral rotation of the thigh. When the extremity is fixed, bilateral contraction causes the trunk to flex, whereas unilateral contraction of the muscle rotates the pelvis and trunk in opposite directions.

Palpatory technique: With the patient supine, the origin is palpated through the abdominal wall, which should be completely relaxed. The promontory is located (correlating to L_5). The fingers then follow the vertebral bodies laterally, reaching the lateral circumference and consequently move superior to L_1 level. The four fingers then move laterally along the vertebral bodies to the muscle belly, and the patient is asked to raise the leg straight up (when myotendinotic changes have occured, painfulness normally increases).

The insertion at the lesser trochanter can also be palpated. Again the patient is supine, and the fingers search the lesser trochanter behind the adductors while the legs are flexed and abducted.

SRS correlation: See table. The psoas major muscle, which supports body posture, tends to shorten and is very often involved in the spondylogenic event (it is possibly correlated with the upper cervical spine). Myotendinosis and muscle shortening can develop as a result of an anteriorly functionally abnormal position of the vertebra. This has to be taken into account when establishing diagnosis and therapy.

7.20. Psoas Minor Muscle

Origin: vertebral bodies of T_{12} and L_1 below the arcuate ligament of the diaphragm.

Insertion: at the pecten ossis pubis, the inguinal ligament (broad junction), and the iliopectineal line (iliopectineal eminence).

The psoas minor muscle is mentioned for the sake of completeness only. It is very difficult to palpate and is of no significance for SRS aspects.

7.21. Iliacus Muscle

Origin: upper margin of the iliac fossa (Fig. **132**).

Insertion: lesser trochanter of femur.

Course and relations: The muscle fibers converge toward the lacuna musculorum (ilium) where they attach to the lateral edge of the psoas major muscle to insert together at the lesser trochanter of the femur.

Innervation and function: same as the psoas major muscle.

Palpatory technique: The iliac muscle can be palpated in the iliac fossa only with difficulty, and then incompletely. In order to relax the abdominal musculature, the patient is brought into a half-sitting position. The thumb reaches around the anterior-superior iliac spine and slides deep along the upper part of the illum. The iliac muscle can be followed along the iliac crest from the anterior iliac spine by going superior for about three finger widths and inferior by two finger widths, at the most. The remaining fibers at the origin cannot be followed distinctly due to their anatomic position and the overlying abdominal musculature.

SRS correlation: See Figure **132**.

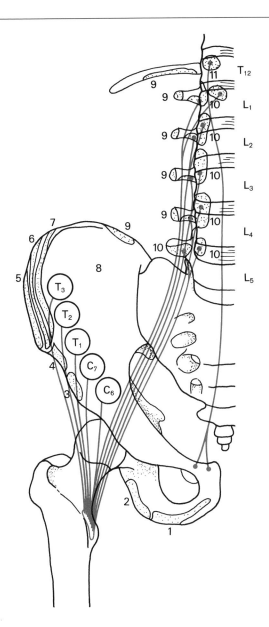

Fig. **132**. Iliopsoas muscle.

1: Adductor magnus m
2: Quadratus femoris m
3: Rectus femoris m
4: Sartorius m
5: External abdominal oblique m
6: Internal abdominal oblique m
7: Transversus abdominis m
8: Iliacus m
9: Quadratus lumborum m
10: Psoas major m
11: Psoas minor m

7.22. Sternocleidomastoid Muscle

This large, rounded muscle passes obliquely across the side of the neck, being twisted 90° about its longitudinal axis in a screw like manner so that its inferior portion is directed anteriorly and its superior portion laterally. At the origin, the tendon of the sternocleidomastoid muscle is divided into a clavicular and a sternal portion. The muscle belly unites to form one strong insertion.

Origin: *Sternal portion:* The muscle arises as a rounded, strong tendon from the anterior surface of the manubrium of the sternum, immediately medial and somewhat inferior to the sternoclavicular joint (Fig. **133**).

Clavicular portion: This portion is composed of both muscular and aponeurotic (tendon) fibers and arises from the superior surface and the posterior border of the sternal end of the clavicle. The origin extends laterally from the joint to the first third of the clavicle. The flat muscle belly slides under the inferior surface of the sternal portion and becomes enlarged superiorly.

Insertion: The muscle inserts into the outer surface of the mastoid process from its tip to its superior border and further to the center of the superior nuchal line (Figs. **133, 134**).

Course and relations: (See Fig. **53**, the cross-section of the cervical spine). The sternocleidomastoid muscle is covered to a great extent by the platysma muscle. From its origin to its insertion, the muscle passes superficially and obliquely across the anterior side of the neck, thereby dividing the neck region in two: the anterior and lateral regions. It would be beyond the scope of this book to cover the topographical importance of these two anatomical triangles in further detail (please refer to anatomy texts).

Innervation: the spinal accessory nerve and partially the cervical plexus (C_2–C_3).

Function: Bilateral contraction results in flexion of the head, and unilateral contraction results in lateral bending of the head to the side of the contracted muscle and rotation to the opposite side.

Palpatory technique: The origin of the sternal portion at the manubrium of the the sternum is palpated superolaterally. One has to remain immediately medial to the sternoclavicular joints. When palpating the clavicular portion, the finger reaches around the posterior margin of the clavicle in a hooklike manner. The homologous insertion tendinoses are palpated at the external surface of the mastoid process, going inferior from its apex to the superior nuchal line.

SRS correlation: The sternocleidomastoid muscle consists of four myotenones, which are correlated with the vertebrae T_4–T_8. Their arrangement can be seen in Figure **133**.

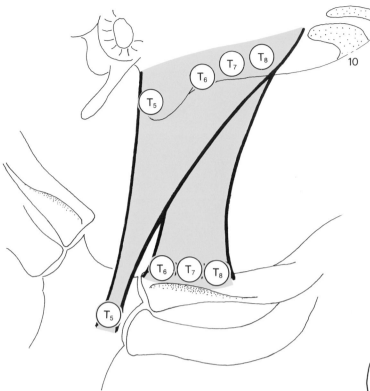

Fig. **133**. Sternocleidomastoid muscle.

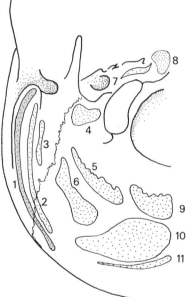

Fig. **134**. Muscle attachment at the occiput.

 1: Sternocleidomastoid m
 2: Splenius capitis m
 3: Longissimus capitis m
 4: Rectus capitis lateralis m
 5: Rectus capitis posterior major m
 6: Obliquus capitis superior m
 7: Rectus capitis anterior m
 8: Longus capitis m
 9: Rectus capitis posterior minor m
10: Semispinalis capitis m
11: Trapezius m
12: Obliquus capitis inferior m

7.23. Deltoid Muscle

Origin: *Clavicular portion:* lateral third of the clavicle. *Acromial portion:* the acromion. *Scapular portion:* from the spine of the scapula.

The most posterior fibers arise from the infraspinatous fascia (Fig. **135**).

Insertion: The muscle inserts at the deltoid tuberosity of the humerus; the relatively small area of insertion has the shape of an escutcheon (Fig. **136**); it passes to the intermuscular septum of the lateral and medial arm.

Course and relations: The broad deltoid muscle covers all muscles inserting at the proximal end of the humerus.

The great difference between the length of the origin (more than 20 cm) and the area of insertion (15 × 15 mm) is responsible for the extensive convergence of the fibers.

Innervation: axillary (circumflex) nerve.

Function: The main function of the muscle is abduction in the shoulder joint, the acromial portion of the muscle being the main abductor.

The clavicular portion is synergistic to the pectoralis major muscle; the scapular portion is synergistic to the latissimus dorsi and teres major muscles.

Palpatory technique: Similar to the gluteal musculature, the deltoid muscle can be palpated directly. Especially the origin tendinoses must be demarcated exactly in the direction of the converging fibers (Fig. **136**). The transitional tendinoses are located at the fibers most posterior, that is, at the transition into the infraspinous fascia. The insertion tendinoses can be defined only theoretically, according to their spondylogenic correlation. The intermuscular septum, however, which is often subject to pain can be palpated practically to its insertion at the lateral epicondyle.

SRS correlation: The SRS correlation, which can only be differentiated at the origin, is reproduced in Figure **135**.

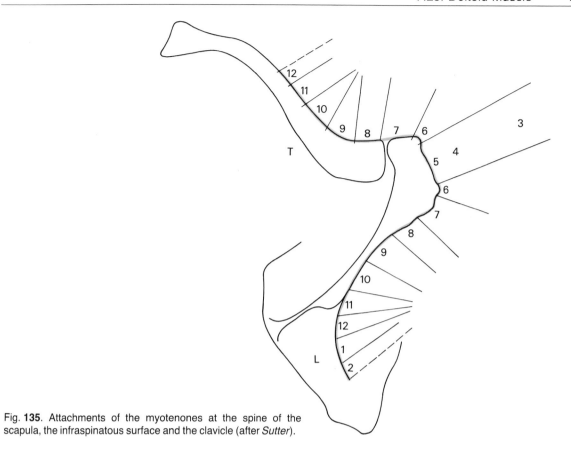

Fig. **135**. Attachments of the myotenones at the spine of the scapula, the infraspinatous surface and the clavicle (after *Sutter*).

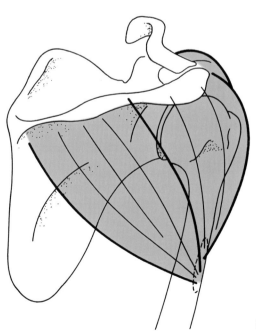

Fig. **136**. Deltoid muscle.

7.24. Gluteus Maximus Muscle

Origin: In the area of origin, the gluteus maximus muscle can be divided into two layers; this fact is of spondylogenic importance (see below).

Superficial layer:
 – From the iliac crest
 – From the posterior superior iliac spine
 – From the thoracolumbar fascia
 – From the lateral sacral line
 – From the coccyx

Deep layer:
 – From the broad, upper portion of the ilium, behind the posterior gluteal line
 – From the sacrotuberous ligament
 – From the fascia covering the gluteus medius (Fig. **137**).

Insertion: The superficial and the deep layers unite in their course. The superior portions pass into the iliotibial tract (tibial portion) at the level of the greater trochanter, and the inferior fibers insert at the gluteal tuberosity of the femur, being about 10 cm long (femoral portion); see the diagram of the pelvis, Figure **147**.

Course and relations: The fibers of the tibial portion pass obliquely in a lateroinferior direction. The strong aponeurotic transition into the iliotibial tract is located at the lateral margin of the greater trochanter (transitional tendinoses). The fibers of the femoral part also pass obliquely lateroinferior; thus, the inferior edge of the muscle crosses the horizontal gluteal sulcus.

Innervation: the inferior gluteal nerve L_5, S_1.

Function: extension of the thigh, adduction and lateral rotation of the femur.

Palpatory technique: See diagram of the pelvis Fig. **147**. The origin tendinoses of the superficial layer can easily be reached, the palpatory direction being lateroinferior. The pressure of palpation is exerted tangentially and is of specific importance at the lateral sacral line in order to avoid confusion with the sacral zones of irritation. Myotendinotic changes are palpated obliquely in the direction of the fibers from the origin to insertion, the aponeurotic transition. Even the less experienced examiner should be able to complete this procedure successfully. Thus, the gluteus maximus mus-

cle is used for teaching and practice purposes. The sacral or lumbar zones of irritation, in contrast, serve for comparison and control. Palpation of the deep layer is performed in the same manner, the only difference being the greater palpatory depth which, however, requires the examiner to be more experienced.

SRS correlation: With abnormal position of the sacral or lumbar vertebrae, the gluteus maximus muscle develops myotendinosis rapidly and consistently. The superior fibers (tibial portion) are correlated with the sacroiliac joint and L_5, the inferior fibers (femoral portion) with the superficial layer of the lumbar spine. The fibers of the lower layer have a possible reflexogenic and spondylogenic relationship to the upper thoracic spine. The arrangement and correlation of individual myotendinoses are depicted clearly in Figure **137**.

7.25. Gluteus Medius Muscle

Origin: The gluteus medius muscle arises from a triangle whose sides are formed by the anterior and posterior gluteal lines and the external lip of the iliac crest.

Insertion: The muscle inserts in the outer surface of the great trochanter (superior, lateroposterior quadrant).

Course and relations: The gluteus medius muscle is fan shaped with its fibers arranged like roof tile (Fig. **138**). Due to this arrangement, a superficial and deep layer can be differentiated in the area of origin both anatomically and spondylogenically; these two layers are also separated from each other by loose connective tissue.

Innervation: superior gluteal nerve L_4–S_1.

Function: The muscle as a whole unit serves for the abduction of the thigh; the anterior portion flexes and rotates the thigh medially; the posterior portion extends and rotates the thigh laterally.

Palpatory technique: The tendinoses as well as the myotendinoses of the superficial layer can be found without difficulty; of importance is the differentiation from the gluteus maximus muscle. For precise palpation as well as to obtain clear information from the patient, the thumb must reach the insertion tendinoses just barely inferior to the iliac crest along the muscle fibers direction (Fig. **138**). Myotendinotic changes can be followed to the insertion at the greater trochanter without any difficulty. The insertions of the deep layer are located at the anterior gluteal line.

SRS correlation: The division of the gluteus medius muscle into two parts is also obvious from the spondylogenic correlation: with abnormal positions (segmental dysfunction) in the cervical spine, the deep layer shows myotendinosis, whereas the superior layer reacts upon segmental dysfunctions in the lumbar spine region (Fig. **138**).

The myotenone L_5 in the superficial layer arises from a characteristic location in a flat groove at the junction of the ascending portion and the horizontal portion of the iliac crest. This groove is not a bony formation, yet it can be palpated very easily. L_1 arises directly medial from the iliac spine pointing in the anteroinferior direction whereas T_{12} arises laterally. When the muscle is well developed, a further myotenone is present, which is correlated with T_{10}.

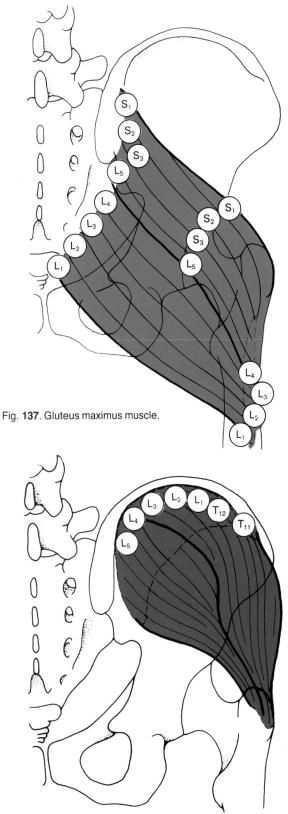

Fig. **137**. Gluteus maximus muscle.

Fig. **138**. Gluteus medius muscle.

7.26. Gluteus Minimus Muscle

Origin: This fan-shaped muscle arises from the outer surface of the ilium, between the inferior and anterior gluteal lines. The posterior fibers arise from the greater sciatic notch (Fig. **139**).

Insertion: anterolateral and superior quadrant of the greater trochanter.

Course and relations: This deep, flat muscle converges toward the greater trochanter and is totally covered by the gluteus medius muscle.

Innervation: superior gluteal nerve L_4–S_1.

Function: abduction of the thigh in addition to the same functions as the gluteal medial muscle.

Palpatory technique: In order to reach the origin of the gluteus minimus muscle, one has to penetrate the gluteus medius and partially the gluteus maximus muscles. The myotendinoses of the origin are palpated along a convex line (pointing slightly superior) from the anterior margin of the ilium to the vicinity of the posterior inferior iliac spine. In practice, palpation is performed from the apex of the trochanter in the direction of the posterior iliac spine, whereby the finger during palpation presses deeply into the soft tissue of the buttocks at different angles.

SRS correlation: The gluteus minimus muscle is correlated spondylogenically with the lower thoracic spine. The arrangement and correlation of the individual myotenones can be seen in Figure **139**.

7.27. Piriformis Muscle

Origin: The anterior surface of the pelvis between the sacral foramina II to IV (Fig. **140**).

Insertion: the superomedial apex of the greater trochanter.

Course and relations: The piriformis muscle passes from the lateral surface of the sacrum to the greater sciatic foramen, thereby leaving the lesser pelvis to insert finally at the greater trochanter (Fig. **141**).

Passing through the greater sciatic foramen the piriformis muscle divides this foramen into superior and inferior portions. This is of great clinical importance, since the piriformis muscle is in close proximity to the sciatic nerve, the inferior gluteal nerve, the posterior cutaneous nerve of the thigh, and the pudendal nerve.

Innervation: rami from the sacral plexus S_1.

Function: lateral rotation of the thigh.

Palpatory technique: The piriformis muscle can be palpated at one particular point in the gluteal region after its exit from the greater sciatic foramen. This point is the intersection of two lines that are constructed as follows: the first line is the connection between the superior posterior iliac spine and the greater trochanter; the other line runs from the anterior superior iliac spine and the lower pole of the coccyx. Myotendinosis of the piriformis muscle can be very painful. In order to eliminate doubt or for further verification, the origin must be examined rectally at the anterior surface of the sacrum (Fig. **141**).

SRS correlation: The piriformis muscle represents one single myotenone that is correlated with L_5.

Remarks: The piriformis muscle is important in posture, and it decidedly tends to shorten. Similar to the psoas major muscle, the piriformis muscle often is involved in the SRS event. Chronic myotendinosis in piriformis muscle can even cause neural symptoms as a result of its anatomical proximity to the sciatic nerve. These symptoms are difficult to differentiate from a discogenic radicular condition.

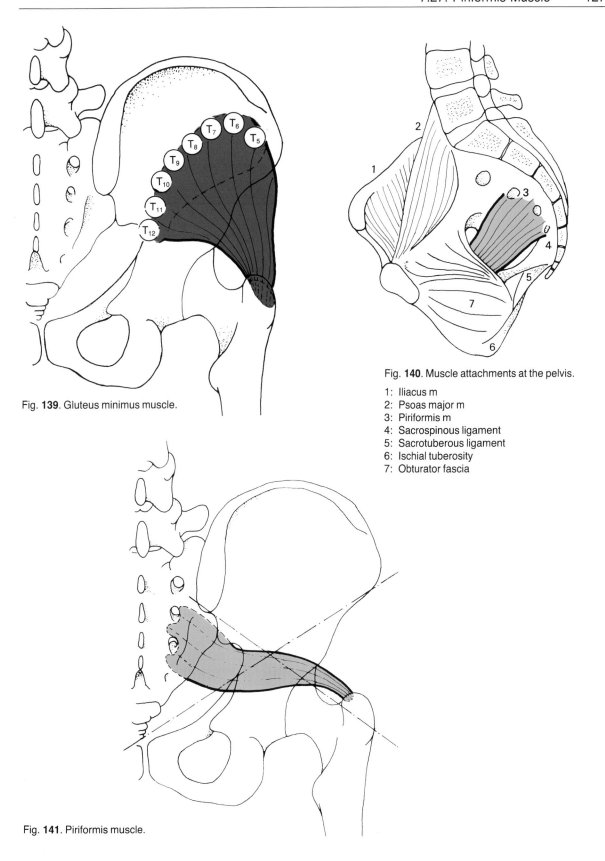

Fig. **139**. Gluteus minimus muscle.

Fig. **140**. Muscle attachments at the pelvis.

1: Iliacus m
2: Psoas major m
3: Piriformis m
4: Sacrospinous ligament
5: Sacrotuberous ligament
6: Ischial tuberosity
7: Obturator fascia

Fig. **141**. Piriformis muscle.

8. Ligaments of the Pelvis

Palpation and differentiation of the individual ligaments is difficult and can even be impossible due to
the anatomical position, such as when involving the
transverse ligament of the atlas, the alar ligaments,
and the anterior sacroiliac ligament. In this chapter, only those ligaments are described that provide
access for clinical palpation and those known for
their significance in SRS and their spondylogenic
correlation.

8.1. Iliolumbar Ligament

Origin: the inferior and lateral margin of the tips of
the costal processes of L_4 and L_5. These two origins
and their corresponding tendons are anatomically
independent of each other in their course (iliac
tuberosity junction) (Fig. **142**).

Insertion: This ligament inserts in the most medial
portions of the iliac crest and the neighboring
anterior and posterior surfaces of the ilium
(Fig. **143**).

Course and relations: As mentioned, the tendons
arising from L_4 and L_5 must be considered sepa-
rately:

L_4-segment: Arising from the costal process of L_4,
this part of the tendon passes steeply inferiorly and
laterally reaching the anterior surface of the ilium
lateral to the sacroiliac joint (Figs. **142, 143**).

L_5-segment: This portion divides in two immediately at the origin of the costal process of L_5
(Figs. **142, 143**).

Fibers arising from the tip pass almost perfectly
horizontally to the iliac tuberosity, reaching the
anterior side of the ilium where they insert together
with the fibers from L_4.

Fibers arising from the costal process of L_5 pass
lateroinferiorly, almost vertically, to the anterior
side of the ilium, reaching the linea terminalis,
where they insert together with the anterior sacroiliac ligaments.

Function: The iliolumbar ligament transmits the
motion of the hip bones to the vertebrae L_4 and L_5.
Thus, it plays an important role in the mechanics of
the lumbopelvic junction.

Palpatory technique: When palpating this anatomically small space, one should be aware that the
iliolumbar ligament lies extremely deep. The fibers
arising from L_4 are still accessible to palpation:
from a laterosuperior direction, the origin at the
costal process is palpated, whereas the insertion is
palpated mediosuperiorily as long as it is accessible
at the iliac crest.

When palpating for the fibers arising from L_5, only
the insertion of the horizontal portion of the fibers
is accessible. Palpation, however, presents clear
results only after the tendon has become painful.

SRS correlation: L_4-segment equals T_4 and T_5.
L_5-segment equals T_6 and T_7.

Remarks: The supportive function of the iliolumbar ligament in the lumbosacral junction is of great
significance. If it is spondylogenically affected, it
can cause intense back pain, especially when raising the trunk from the flexed position. This
ligamentous pain is often persistent and resistant to
therapy. Patients complain about diffused back
pain when either in the flexed or extended position
(such as vacuuming or ironing).

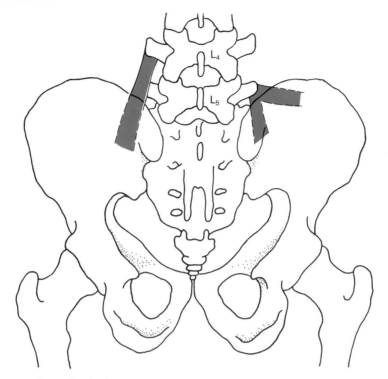

Fig. **142**. Iliolumbar ligament (posterior view).

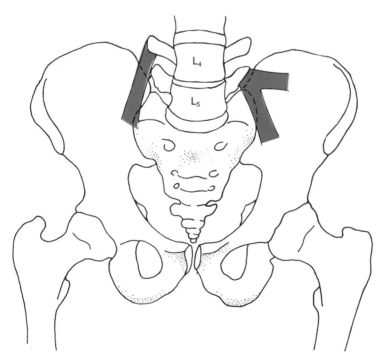

Fig. **143**. Iliolumbar ligament (anterior view).

8.2. Sacrospinous Ligament

Origin: the side of the coccyx and the entire free sacrum up to the level of S_3.

Insertion: the spine of the ischium (apex and superior margin). The line of insertion is quite narrow (about 1 cm).

Course and relations: The sacrospinous ligament lies anterior to the sacrotuberous ligament. Both ligaments interdigitate at their origin at the free margin of the sacrum. Constructing a vertical line through the posterior superior iliac spine, one meets the spine of the ischium inferiorly at the level of the sacrococcyxgeal junction. From this constructed landmark, the fan-shaped sacrospinous ligament passes to the sacrum and coyycx, that is, in medial to superomedial direction whereby the most inferior fibers are almost horizontal. Laterally, the ligament underlies the muscle mass of the gluteus maximus muscle and medially it is only covered by the thin lining of the abdominal cavity.

Palpatory technique: The origin of the sacrospinous ligament is covered by the origin of the gluteus maximus muscle. Thus, with incorrect palpatory depth one can confuse this ligament with the tendinoses of the superficial gluteus maximus layer. The origin can be reached from lateral (bony contact) without any major difficulty. This origin is palpated through the musculature of the gluteus muscle at the correct topographical location (see before) from a posterior direction.

Rectal examination, however, is far superior to external palpation and is the method of choice, especially when definitive clarification becomes necessary.

SRS correlation: The sacrospinous ligament is spondylogenically correlated with the cervical spine; fibers arising most inferiorly at the origin (margin of the coccyx-sacrum) are correlated with the C_0 segment; fibers arising from the most superior portion are correlated with the segment C_6 (Fig. **144**).

It is practically impossible to differentiate individual tendinoses at the spine of the ischium due to the narrow field of insertion.

Remarks: The sacrospinous ligament is of great spondylogenic, and clinical importance. Often a persistent coccydynia can be caused by the sacrospinous ligament as a result of a functional disturbance in the upper cervical spine region, for instance.

Myotendinosis in the superior fibers can cause a S_1-dysfunction, whereas myotendinosis in the inferior fiber tracts can cause dysfunction in S_2.

The sacrospinous ligament shows great anatomical variation. Different portions of varying size can develop into contractile muscle fibers, and in very rare cases, the whole tendon can form the coccygeal muscle. In regard to the spondylogenic correlation, it is insignificant whether it is tendon or muscle. Considering the phenomenon of "myotendinosis," no fundamental difference exists between the muscular and ligamentous forms. This fact demonstrates that myotendinosis does not necessarily require myofibril contractility.

8.3. Posterior Sacroiliac Ligament

Origin: This ligament arises as a small band from the posterior surface of the sacrum at the level of S_3 and S_4, between the lateral sacral crest and the sacral foramina. Fibers that arise most laterally intermingle with the fibers of the sacrotuberous ligament, whose origin is at this location as well.

Insertion: The tendon inserts along the entire width (about 1 to 2 cm) of the inferior margin of the posterior superior iliac spine (see Palpatory Technique).

Course and relations: The posterior sacroiliac ligament passes almost vertically from its origin at the sacrum to its insertion at the posterior superior iliac spine. The lateral portions of the tendon are in anatomical proximity to the sacrotuberous ligaments, the medial portions to the thoracolumbar fascia (Fig. **145**).

Palpatory technique: The tendon is located in a groove formed by the insertion of the gluteus maximus muscle and the insertion of the sacrospinous system. Due to this anatomical arrangement, few structures overlie the tendon.

It is possible to misidentify this tendon for the sacral zones of irritation, the origin tendinoses of the longissimus thoracis muscle (sector II), and the

(Continued p. 132)

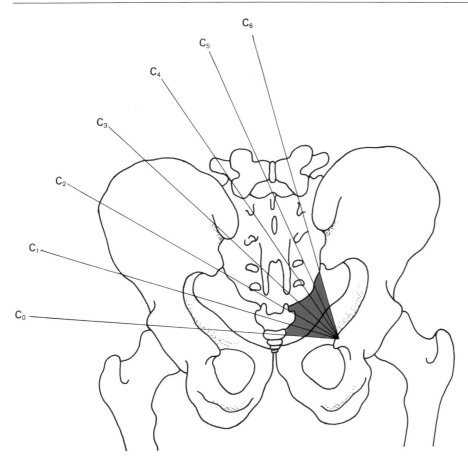

Fig. **144**. Sacrospinous ligament.

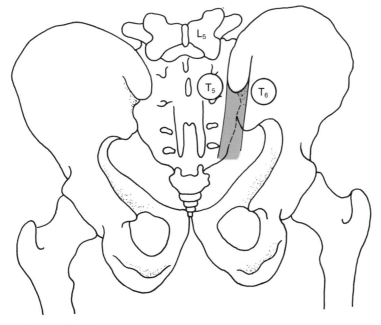

Fig. **145**. Long posterior sacroiliac ligament.

8.4.   Sacrotuberous Ligament

Origin: The sacrotuberous ligament arises above the sacrospinous ligament at the coccyx and the free margin of the side of the sacrum. In contrast to the sacrospinous ligament, the insertion of the sacrotuberous ligament passes further superiorly, reaching the posterior inferior spine; it also joins the fascia lata.

Insertion: From its insertion at the inner surface of the ischial tuberosity a segment of the tendon continues anteriorly along the inner margin of the ramus of the ischium to the posterior margin of the symphysis, forming the so-called falciform ligament. Thus, the insertion is about 5 to 6 cm long.

Course and relations: The sacrotuberous ligament has a fan-shaped appearance. Its fibers pass in a propeller-like fashion from origin to insertion. Thus, the fiber tracts undergo a changeover with fibers arising most superiorly, cutting across anteromedially (practically vertical) and inserting at the ramus of the ischium most anteriorly. Fibers arising at the most inferior portion, in contrast, ascend posterolaterally to the ischial tuberosity, reaching the line of insertion at the most posterior portion (Fig. **146**).

The sacrotuberous ligament lies posterior to the sacrospinous ligament, which is weaker and shorter.

Portions of the sacrotuberous ligament close to the origin serve as origin for a great part of the gluteus maximus muscle.

Palpatory technique: When palpating the origin (at the coccyx, sacrum) one has to be aware of the anatomical relationship of the sacrotuberous ligament to the sacrospinous ligament and the gluteus maximus muscle. The sacral zones of irritation lie more medial and should not be the cause of confusion. Palpation follows the muscle fiber direction from lateral to the margin of the sacrum. In the prone position it should not be difficult to palpate the ischial tuberosity. Starting from the ischial tuberosity, insertion tendinoses are then located by palpating along the ramus of the ischium to the posterior margin of the symphysis (the falciform ligament.) Rectal examination may again become necessary.

SRS correlation: The sacrotuberous ligament is spondylogically correlated with the upper thoracic spine (C_7 to T_8). The propeller-like arrangement of the fibers finds its expression in the SRS correlation and its manifestation, as seen in Figure **146**.

Remarks: Similar to remarks made for the sacrospinous ligament. Myotendinosis of the superior fibers favors S_1 disturbances, whereas myotendinosis of the inferior fibers favors S_2 disturbances.

(p. 130 continued)

most inferior origins of the transverospinous system. The insertion at the posterior superior iliac spine is of practical importance for palpation; this insertion is palpated inferiorly and slightly medially in the direction of the posterior superior iliac spine.

SRS correlation: The posterior sacroiliac ligament is correlated with the SRS of T_5 and T_6. Whether the tendon participates in the spondylogenic event is determined by considering the insertion at the posterior superior iliac spine. At this location, the fibers correlating to T_5 lie medial to the posterior superior iliac spine (inferior margin) and fibers correlating to T_6 lie lateral to the posterior superior iliac spine (Fig. **145**).

Remarks: Due to the anatomical arrangement, myotendinosis in the posterior sacroiliac ligaments can cause an abnormal position of S_3.

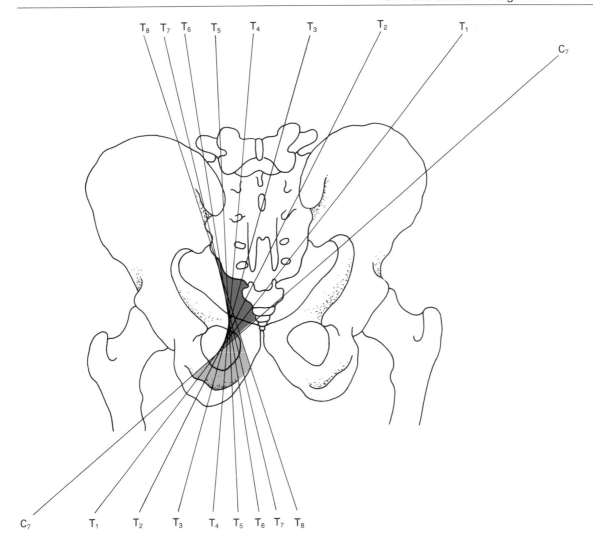

Fig. **146**. Sacrotuberous ligament.

9. Overview of Important Tendinoses and Zones of Irritation in the Lumbar-Pelvic Region

(Fig. 147)

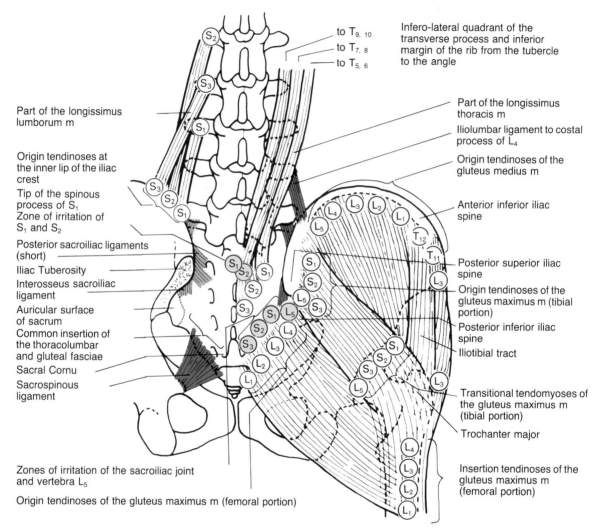

to $T_{9,\ 10}$
to $T_{7,\ 8}$
to $T_{5,\ 6}$

Infero-lateral quadrant of the transverse process and inferior margin of the rib from the tubercle to the angle

Part of the longissimus lumborum m

Origin tendinoses at the inner lip of the iliac crest

Tip of the spinous process of S_1
Zone of irritation of S_1 and S_2

Posterior sacroiliac ligaments (short)

Iliac Tuberosity

Interosseus sacroiliac ligament

Auricular surface of sacrum

Common insertion of the thoracolumbar and gluteal fasciae

Sacral Cornu

Sacrospinous ligament

Part of the longissimus thoracis m

Iliolumbar ligament to costal process of L_4

Origin tendinoses of the gluteus medius m

Anterior inferior iliac spine

Posterior superior iliac spine

Origin tendinoses of the gluteus maximus m (tibial portion)

Posterior inferior iliac spine

Iliotibial tract

Transitional tendomyoses of the gluteus maximus m (tibial portion)

Trochanter major

Insertion tendinoses of the gluteus maximus m (femoral portion)

Zones of irritation of the sacroiliac joint and vertebra L_5

Origin tendinoses of the gluteus maximus m (femoral portion)

Fig. **147**. (after *Sutter* and *Oberli*).

10. Atlas of the Individual Spondylogenic Reflex Syndromes

Only the most important myotendinoses of isolated SRS are represented. Depending upon the extent of the SRS, the muscles represented can take part in the complete appearance of SRS, but do not necessarily have to do so. In practice, we most often find a mixture of two, three, or more SRSs, causing certain diagnostic difficulties at the beginning of treatment. This is due to the fact that reflexogenically inititated myotendinosis of a myotenone can bring those vertebrae into abnor-

mal position at which it inserts. This abnormal position, in turn, can cause another myotendinosis of those myotenones, which are spondylogenically related to it.

All abnormal positions (segmental dysfunctions) that have been elicited must be treated. After two or three treatments, the original problem is less obscure and is represented as mixed myotendinoses.

**Myotendinoses
(= Myotenones) in the:**

C_0

Thoracic intertransverse m

1   Interspinous ligament

2   Supraspinous ligament

1   Levator costae brevis m

Rotatores muscles

2   Multifidus m.

Semispinalis lumborum m

Psoas major m

✳   Zone of irritations

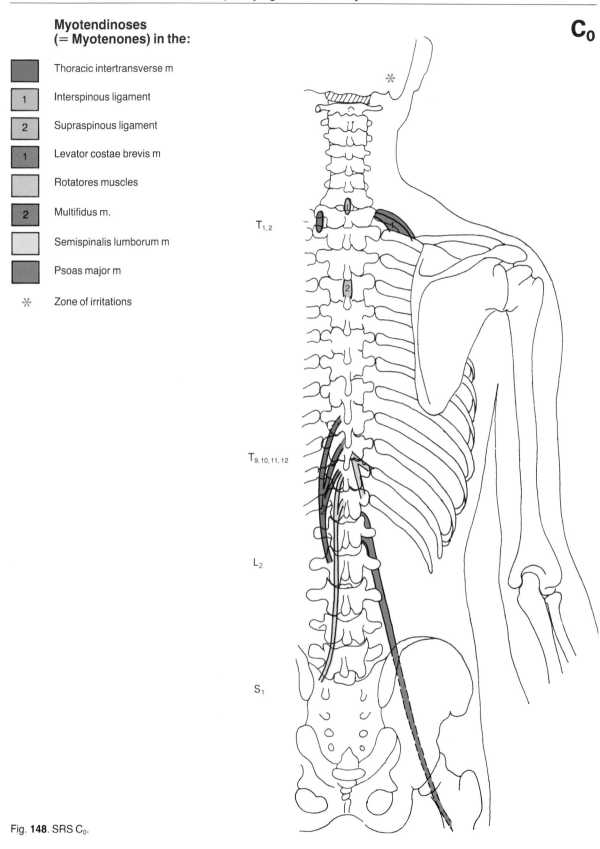

$T_{1,2}$

$T_{9,10,11,12}$

L_2

S_1

Fig. **148**. SRS C_0.

**Myotendinoses
(= Myotenones) in the:**

C₁

1	Anterior cervical intertransverse m
2	Thoracic intertransverse m
1	Interspinous ligament
2	Supraspinous ligament
1	Levator costae brevis m
	Rotatores muscles
2	Multifidus m
	Semispinalis lumborum m
	Psoas major m
	Gluteus medius m (deep layer)
	Latissimus dorsi m
✳	Zone of irritation

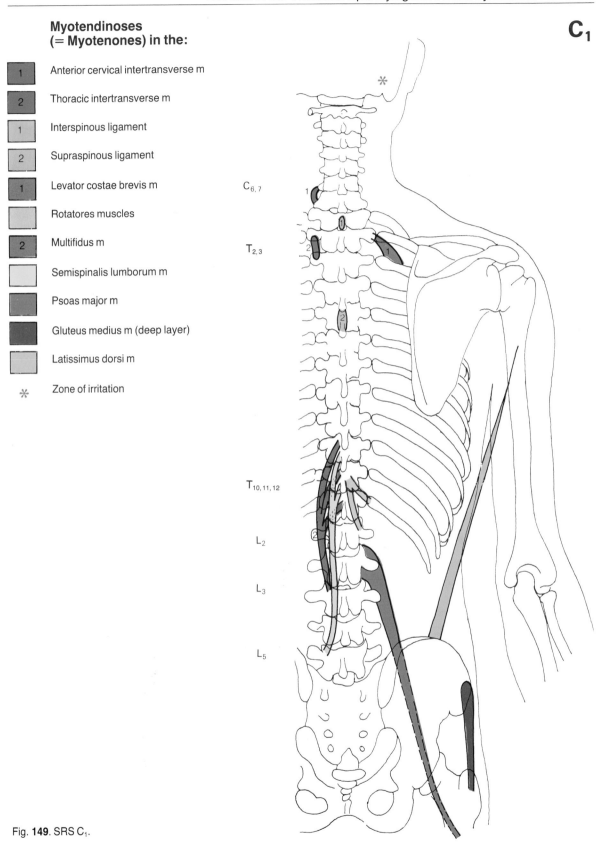

Fig. **149**. SRS C₁.

**Myotendinoses
(= Myotenones) in the:**

C_2

1	Anterior cervical intertransverse m
2	Thoracic intertransverse ligament
1	Interspinous ligament
2	Supraspinous ligament
1	Levator costae brevis m
	Rotatores muscles
2	Multifidus m
	Semispinalis lumborum m
	Psoas major m
	Gluteus medius m (deep layer)
	Latissimus dorsi m
*	Zone of irritation

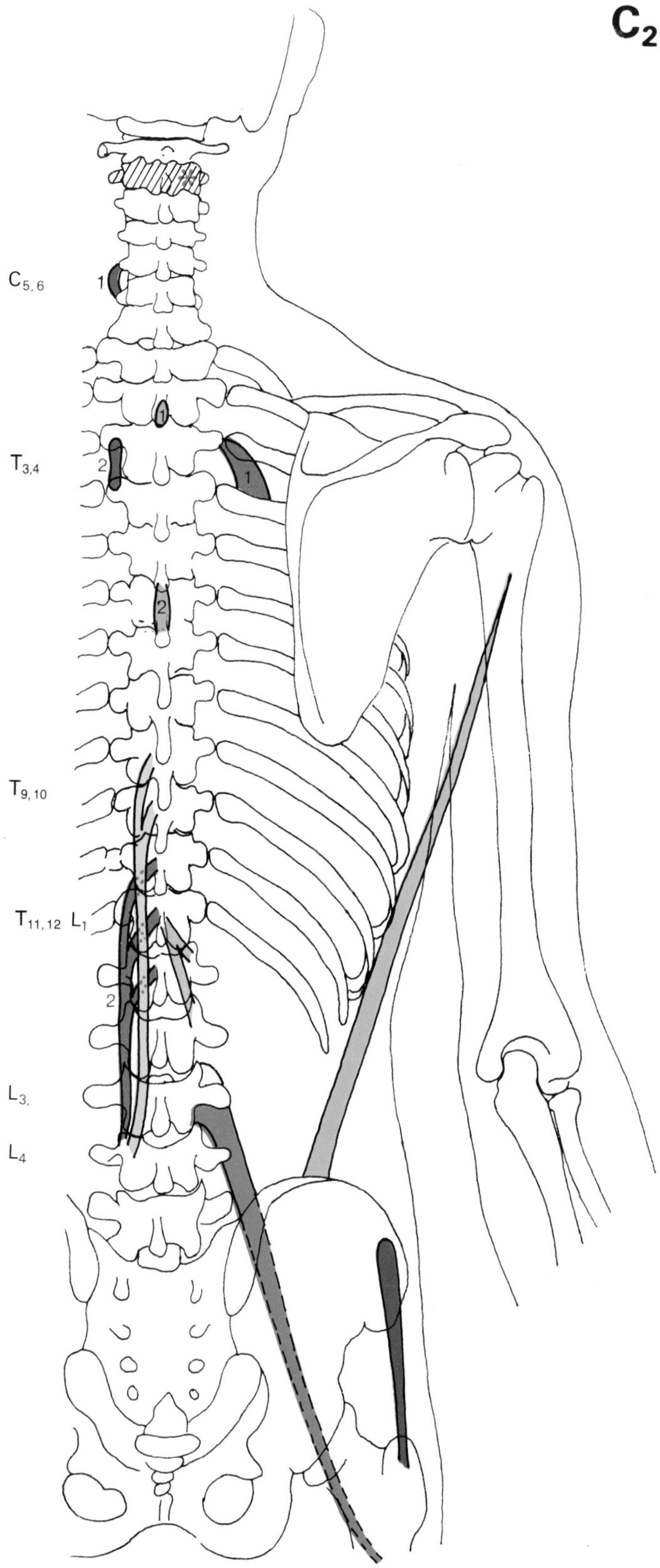

$C_{5,6}$ 1

$T_{3,4}$ 2 1

$T_{9,10}$

$T_{11,12}$ L_1 2

L_3.

L_4

Fig. **150**. SRS C_2.

**Myotendinoses
(= Myotenones) in the:**

C₃

1	Anterior cervical intertransverse m
2	Thoracic intertransverse ligament
1	Interspinous ligament
2	Supraspinous ligament
1	Levator costae brevis m
	Rotatores muscles
2	Multifidus m
	Semispinalis lumborum m
	Psoas major m
	Gluteus medius m (superficial layer)
	Latissimus dorsi m
✳	Zone of irritation

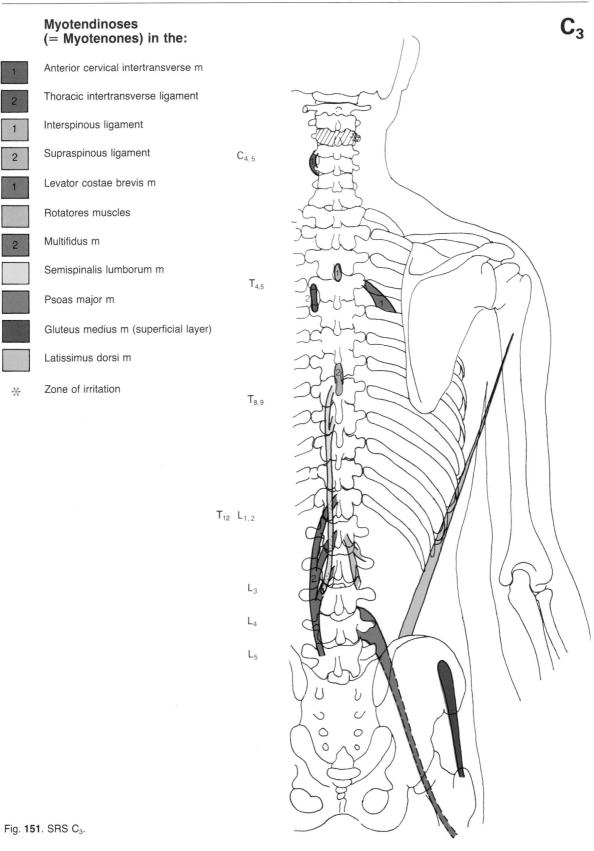

Fig. **151**. SRS C₃.

Myotendinoses
(= Myotenones) in the:

C₄

1	Anterior cervical intertransverse m
2	Thoracic intertransverse ligament
1	Interspinous ligament
2	Supraspinous ligament
1	Levator costae brevis m
	Rhomboid minor m
	Rotatores muscles
2	Multifidus m
	Semispinalis lumborum m
	Psoas major m
	Gluteus medius m (superficial layer)
	Latissimus dorsi m
✳	Zone of irritation

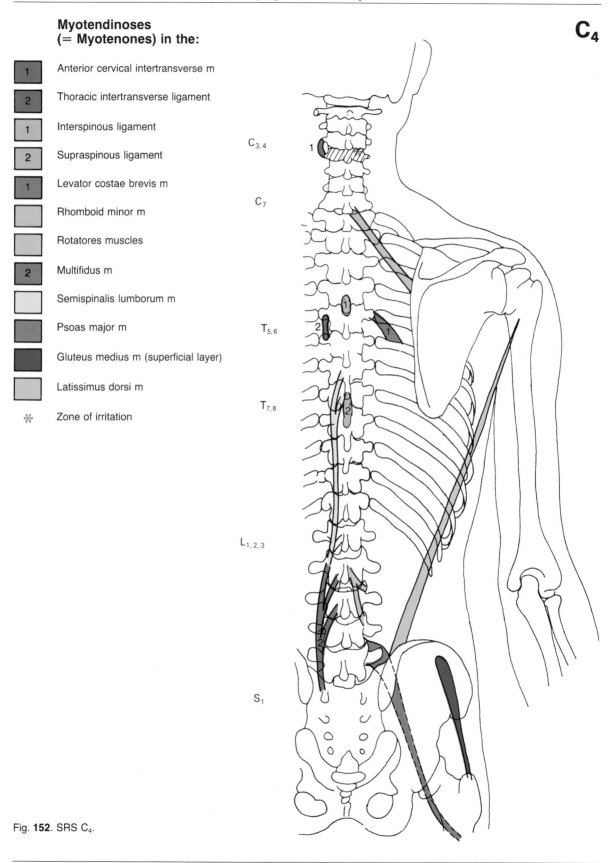

Fig. **152**. SRS C₄.

**Myotendinoses
(= Myotenones) in the:**

C_5

1	Anterior cervical intertransverse m
2	Thoracic intertransverse ligament
1	Interspinous ligament $\quad C_{2,3}$
2	Supraspinous ligament
1	Levator costae brevis m
	Rhomboid major m $\quad T_1$
	Rotatores muscles
2	Multifidus m
	Semispinalis lumborum m
3	Quadratus lumborum m (superficial layer)
	Gluteus medius m (superficial layer) $\quad T_{6,7}$
	Latissimus dorsi m
∗	Zone of irritation

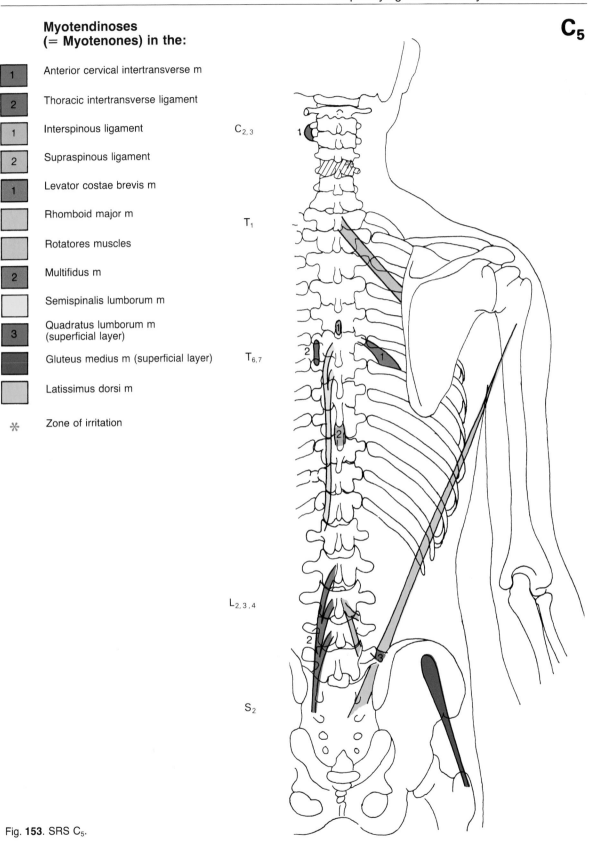

Fig. **153**. SRS C_5.

Myotendinoses
(= Myotenones) in the:

C₆

1	Anterior cervical intertransverse m
2	Thoracic intertransverse ligament
1	Interspinous ligament
2	Supraspinous ligament
1	Levator costae brevis m
	Rhomboid major m
	Rotatores muscles
2	Multifidus m
	Semispinalis lumborum m
3	Quadratus lumborum m (superficial layer)
	Gluteus medius m (superficial layer)
	Latissimus dorsi m
✳	Zone of irritation

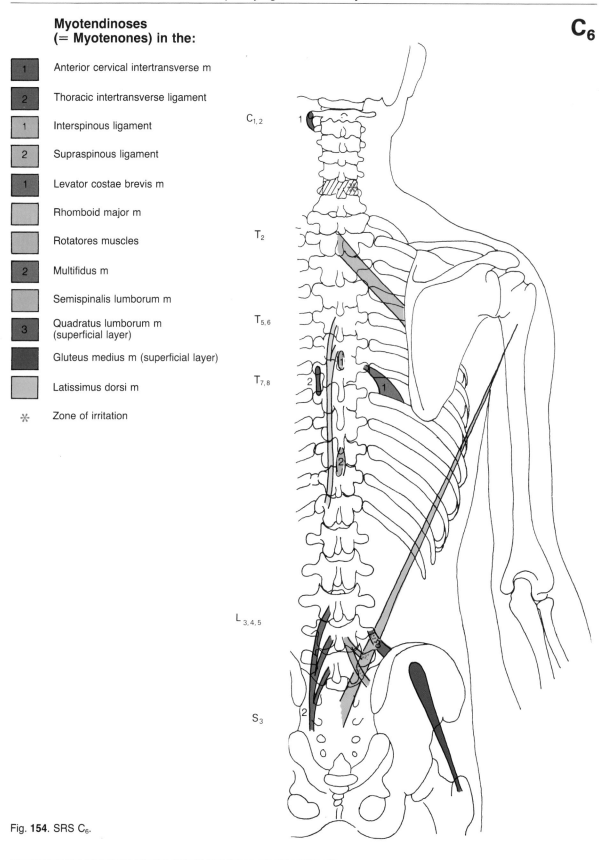

$C_{1,2}$

T_2

$T_{5,6}$

$T_{7,8}$

$L_{3,4,5}$

S_3

Fig. **154**. SRS C₆.

**Myotendinoses
(= Myotenones) in the:**

C_7

1	Anterior rectus capitis m
1	Thoracic intertransverse ligament
1	Interspinalis m and interspinous ligament
2	Supraspinous ligament
2	Levator costae brevis m
1	Rhomboid major m
	Rotatores muscles
3	Multifidus m
	Semispinalis lumborum m
	Longissimus cervicis m
2	Longissimus capitis m
2	Quadratus lumborum m (superficial layer)
	Gluteus medius m (deep layer)
	Latissimus dorsi m
✳	Zone of irritation

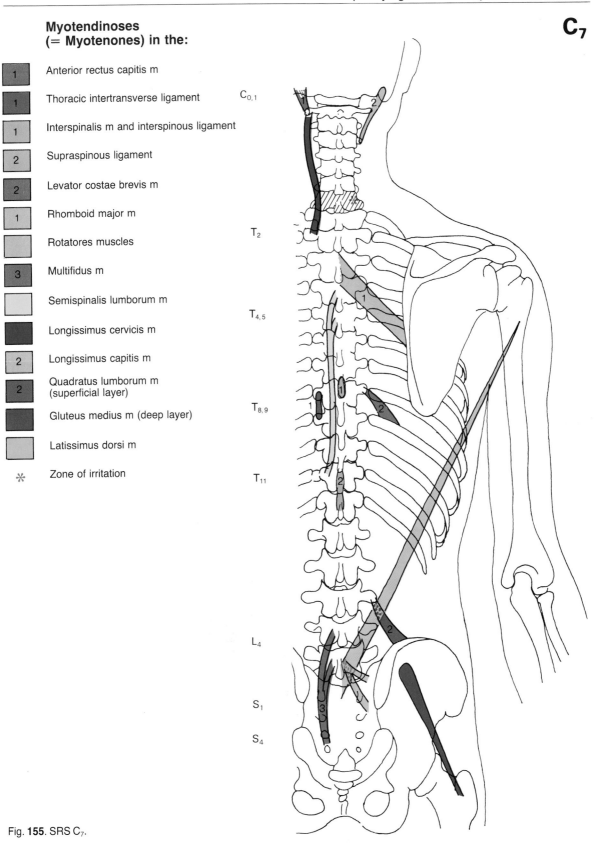

Fig. **155**. SRS C_7.

**Myotendinoses
(= Myotenones) in the:**

T_1

1	Thoracic intertransverse ligament
	Lateralis lumborum intertransverse m
1	Interspinalis m and interspinous ligament
2	Supraspinous ligament
1	Trapezius m (descending portion) (insertion tendinosis)
1	Multifidus m
2	Semispinalis thoracis m
1	Longissimus lumborum m (medial head)
1	Longissimus capitis m
	Longissimus cervicis m
2	Latissimus dorsi m
2	Rhomboid major m
2	Levator costae brevis m
2	Quadratus lumborum m (superficial layer)
✳	Zone of irritation

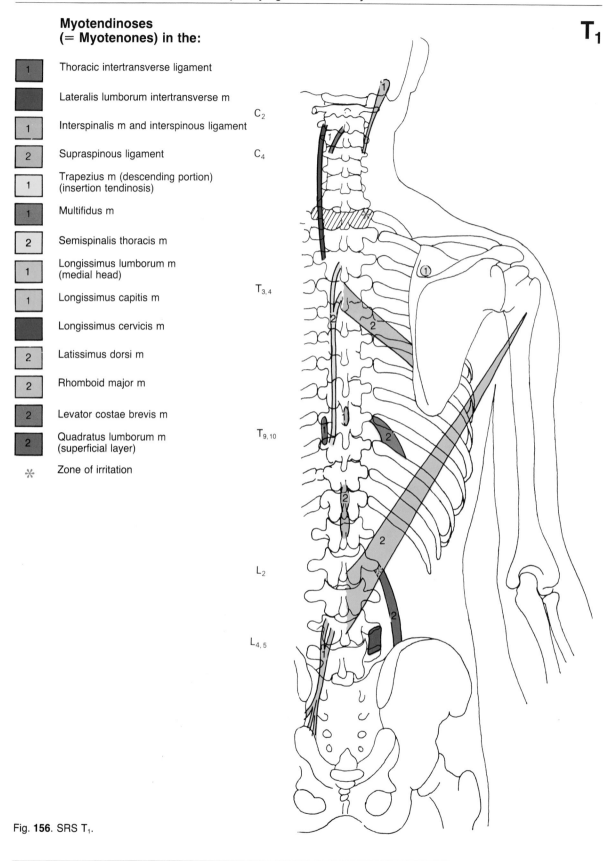

Fig. **156**. SRS T_1.

**Myotendinoses
(= Myotenones) in the:**

T_2

1	Thoracic intertransverse m
	Lateralis lumborum intertransverse m
1	Interspinalis m and interspinous ligament
2	Supraspinous ligament
1	Trapezius m (descending portion) (insertion tendinosis)
	Rotator brevis m
1	Multifidus m
2	Semispinalis thoracis m
1	Longissimus lumborum m (medial head)
1	Longissimus capitis m
	Longissimus cervicis m
2	Latissimus dorsi m
2	Middle scalene m
2	Rhomboid major m
3	Levator scapulae m
2	Levator costae brevis m
3	Quadratus lumborum m (superficial layer)
✳	Zone of irritation

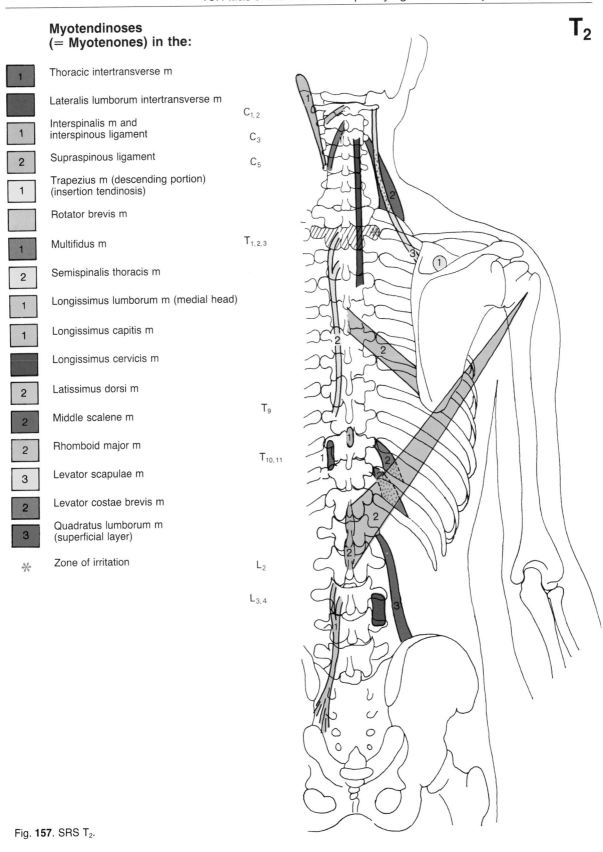

Fig. **157**. SRS T_2.

**Myotendinoses
(= Myotenones) in the:**

T_3

1	Thoracic intertransverse m
	Lateralis lumborum intertransverse m
1	Interspinalis m and interspinous ligament
2	Supraspinous ligament
1	Trapezius m (descending portion) (insertion tendinosis)
	Rotatores muscles
1	Multifidus m
2	Semispinalis thoracis m
1	Longissimus lumborum m (medial head)
	Longissimus capitis m
	Longissimus cervicis m
2	Latissimus dorsi m
2	Middle scalene m
3	Levator scapulae m
2	Levator costae brevis m
✳	Zone of irritation

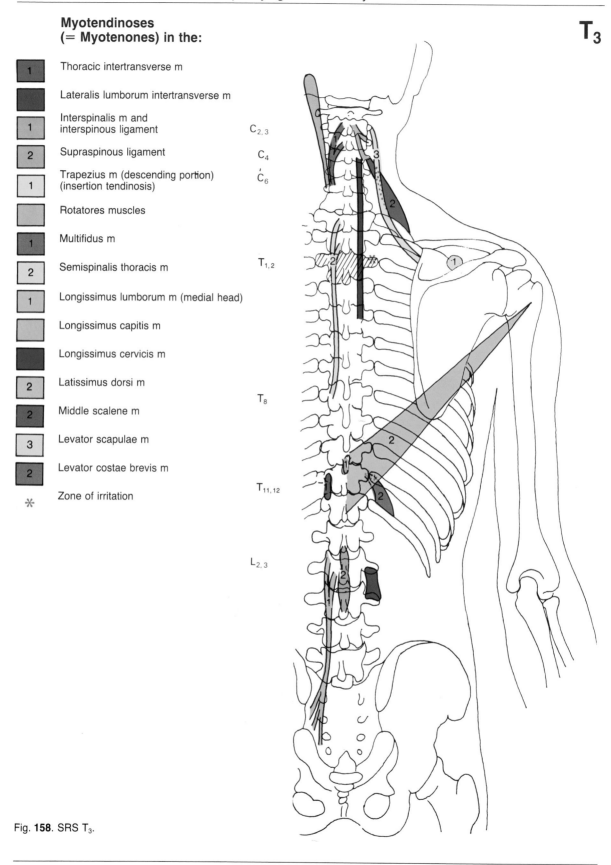

Fig. **158**. SRS T_3.

**Myotendinoses
(= Myotenones) in the:**

T_4

1	Thoracic intertransverse m
1	Lateralis lumborum intertransverse m
1	Interspinalis m and interspinous ligament
2	Supraspinous ligament
1	Semispinalis capitis m
1	Trapezius m (descending portion) (insertion tendinosis)
	Rotatores muscles
2	Multifidus m
2	Semispinalis thoracis m
	Longissimus capitis m
	Longissimus cervicis m
	Latissimus dorsi m
3	Anterior scalene m
2	Middle scalene m
3	Levator scapulae m
3	Iliolumbar ligament
2	Gluteus minimus m
*	Zone of irritation

$C_{2,3,4,5}$

C_7, T_1

T_7

T_{12}

$L_{1,2}$

L_4

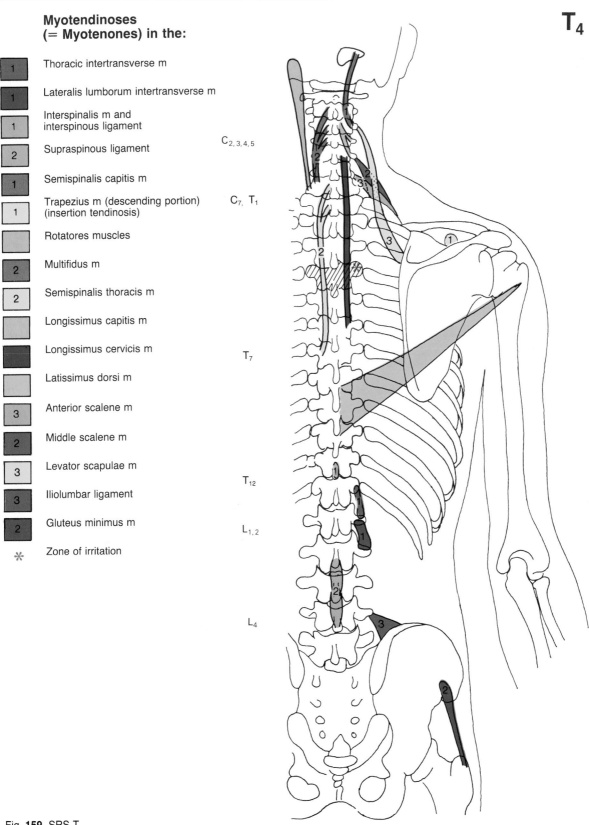

Fig. **159**. SRS T_4.

**Myotendinoses
(= Myotenones) in the:**

T_5

1	Medial lumbar intertransverse m
2	Lateral lumbar intertransverse m
1	Interspinalis m and interspinous ligament
2	Supraspinous ligament
1	Semispinalis capitis m
1	Trapezius m (descending portion) (insertion tendinosis)
	Rotatores muscles
2	Multifidus m
2	Semispinalis cervicis m
	Longissimus thoracis m (sector V)
	Longissimus capitis m
3	Anterior scalene m
1	Middle scalene m
3	Levator scapulae m
2	Iliolumbar ligament
3	Gluteus minimus m
✳	Zone of irritation

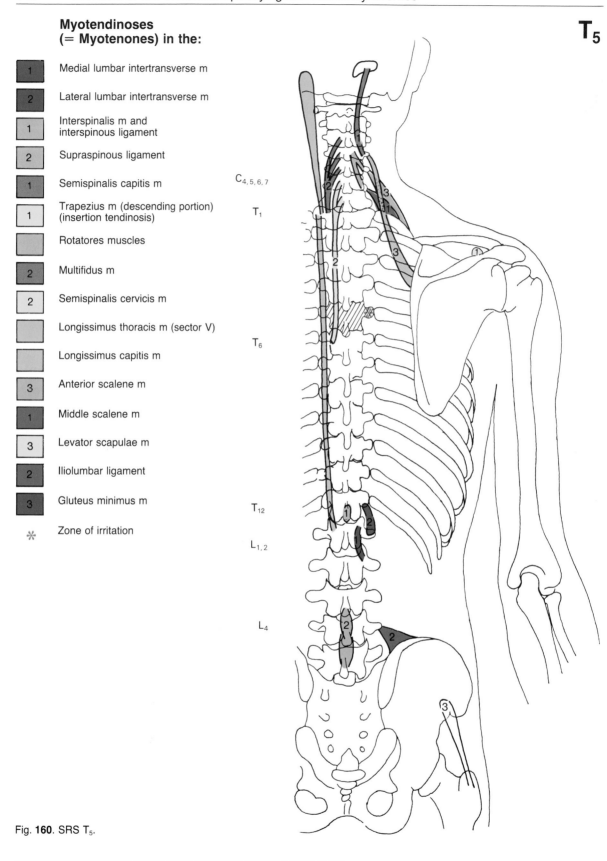

Fig. **160**. SRS T_5.

**Myotendinoses
(= Myotenones) in the:**

T$_6$

1	Medial lumbar intertransverse m
2	Lateral lumbar intertransverse m
1	Interspinalis m and interspinous ligament
2	Supraspinous ligament
1	Semispinalis capitis m
1	Trapezius m (descending portion) (insertion tendinosis)
	Rotatores muscles
2	Multifidus m
2	Semispinalis cervicis m
	Longissimus thoracis m (sector V)
	Longissimus capitis m
3	Anterior scalene m
1	Middle scalene m
2	Iliolumbar ligament
3	Gluteus minimus m
✳	Zone of irritation

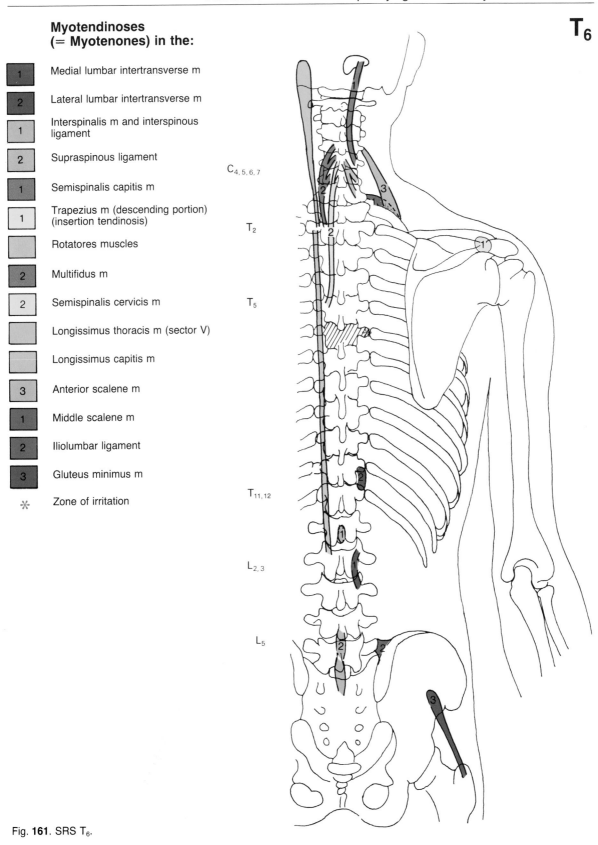

Fig. **161**. SRS T$_6$.

Myotendinoses
(= Myotenones) in the:

T_7

1	Medial lumbar intertransverse m
1	Interspinalis m and interspinous ligament
2	Supraspinous ligament
1	Semispinalis capitis m
1	Trapezius m (descending portion) (insertion tendinosis) $\quad C_{4,5,6,7}$
	Rotatores muscles $\quad T_1$
2	Multifidus m
2	Semispinalis cervicis m $\quad T_{3,4}$
	Longissimus thoracis m (sector V)
	Longissimus capitis m
3	Anterior scalene m
1	Posterior scalene m
2	Iliolumbar ligament
2	Gluteus minimus m
✳	Zone of irritation

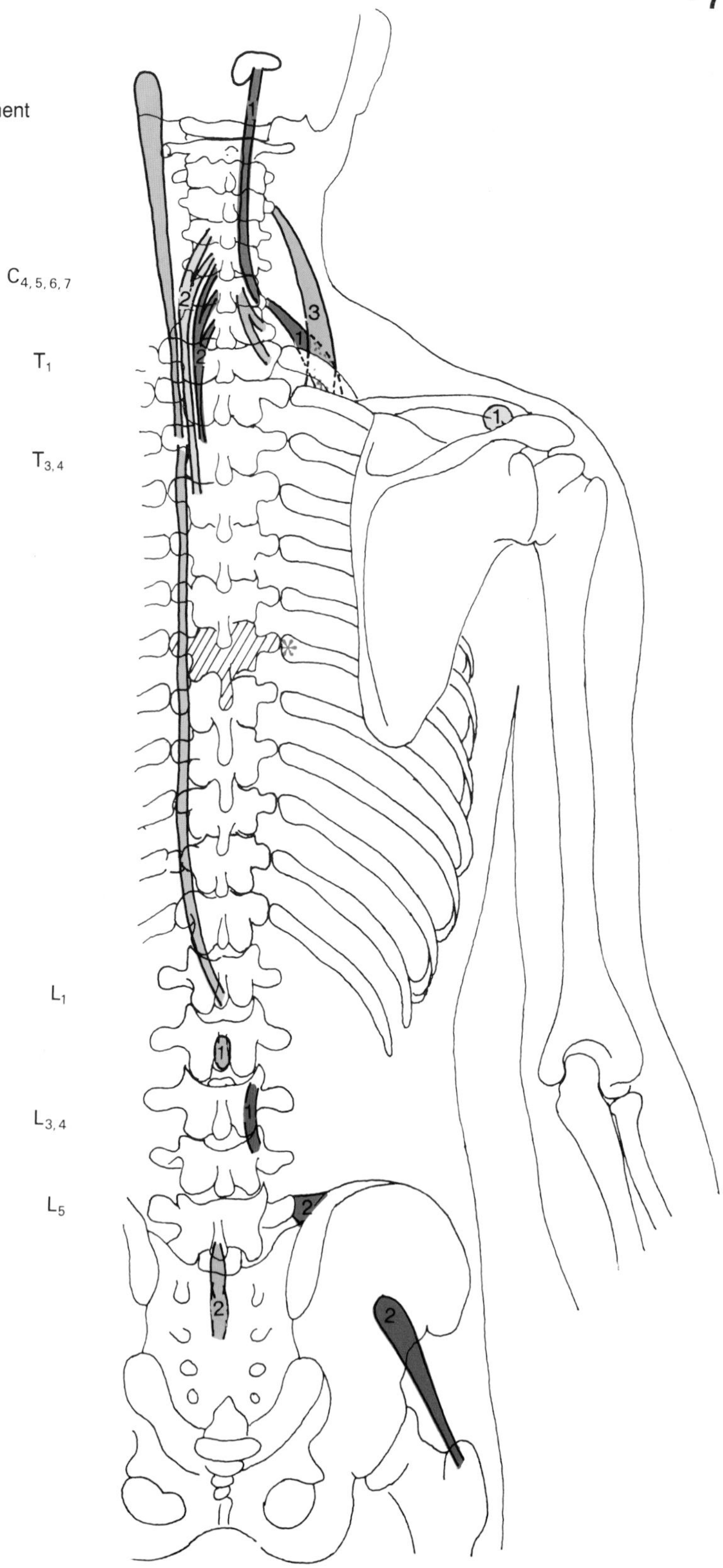

L_1

$L_{3,4}$

L_5

Fig. **162**. SRS T_7.

Myotendinoses
(= Myotenones) in the:

T_8

1	Medial lumbar intertransverse m
1	Interspinalis m and interspinous ligament
2	Supraspinous ligament
1	Semispinalis capitis m
1	Trapezius m (descending portion) (insertion tendinosis)
	Rotatores muscles
2	Multifidus m
2	Semispinalis cervicis m
	Longissimus thoracis m (sector V)
	Longissimus capitis m
	Posterior scalene m
	Quadratus lumborum m (deep layer)
2	Gluteus minimus m
✳	Zone of irritation

$C_{3,4}$

$C_{6,7}$

$T_{3,4}$

$T_{1,2}$

$L_{1,2}$

$L_{4,5}$

S_3

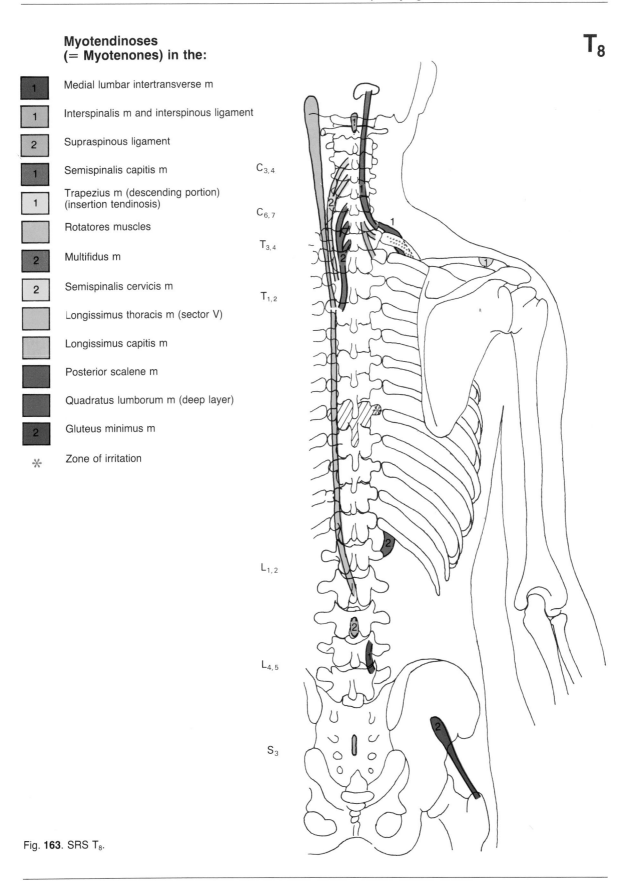

Fig. **163**. SRS T_8.

**Myotendinoses
(= Myotenones) in the:**

T_9

Posterior cervical intertransverse m
(lateral portion)

1 Medial lumbar intertransverse m

1 Interspinalis m and
   interspinous ligament

2 Supraspinous ligament

1 Semispinalis capitis m

1 Trapezius m (descending portion)
   (insertion tendinosis)

Rotatores muscles

2 Multifidus m

2 Semispinalis cervicis m

Longissimus thoracis m (sector II)

Longissimus capitis m

Quadratus lumborum m (deep layer)

2 Gluteus minimus m

✳ Zone of irritation

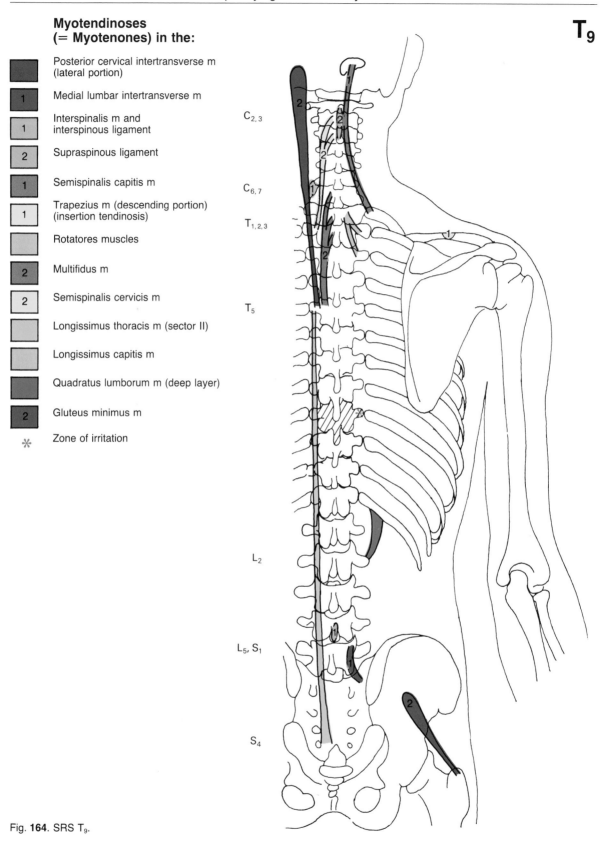

$C_{2,3}$

$C_{6,7}$

$T_{1,2,3}$

T_5

L_2

L_5, S_1

S_4

Fig. **164**. SRS T_9.

Myotendinoses (= Myotenones) in the:

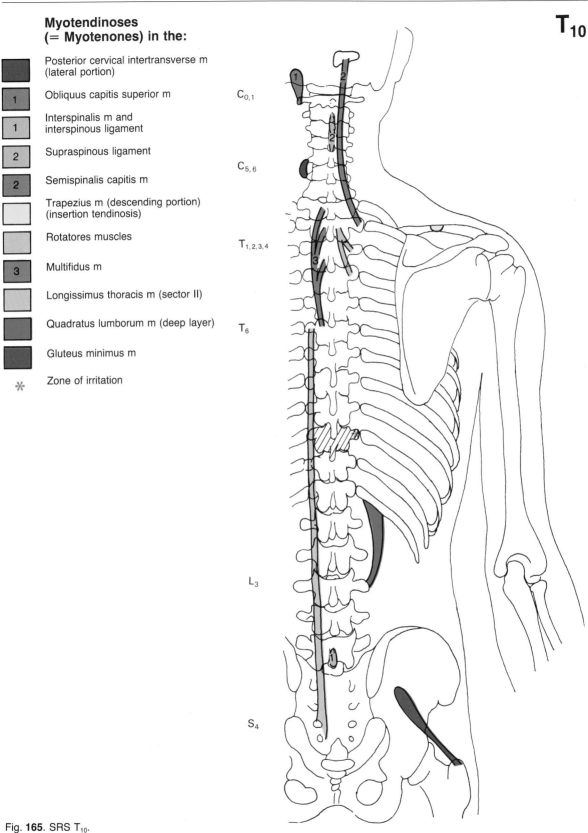

Posterior cervical intertransverse m (lateral portion)

Obliquus capitis superior m $C_{0,1}$

Interspinalis m and **interspinous ligament**

Supraspinous ligament $C_{5,6}$

Semispinalis capitis m

Trapezius m (descending portion) (insertion tendinosis)

Rotatores muscles $T_{1,2,3,4}$

Multifidus m

Longissimus thoracis m (sector II)

Quadratus lumborum m (deep layer) T_6

Gluteus minimus m

* **Zone of irritation**

T_{10}

L_3

S_4

Fig. **165**. SRS T_{10}.

**Myotendinoses
(= Myotenones) in the:**

T_{11}

1 Posterior cervical intertransverse m
(lateral portion)

2 Posterior cervical intertransverse m
(medial portion)

1 Interspinalis m and
interspinous ligament

2 Supraspinous ligament

1 Semispinalis capitis m

Trapezius m (descending portion)
(insertion tendinosis)

Rotatores muscles

2 Multifidus m

Longissimus thoracis m (sector II)

Quadratus lumborum m (deep layer)

Gluteus minimus m

* Zone of irritation

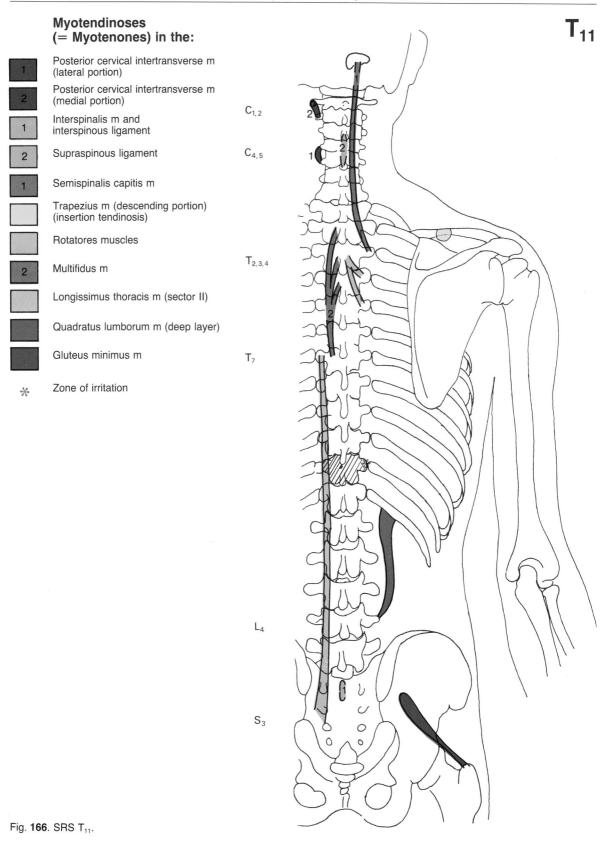

Fig. **166**. SRS T_{11}.

Myotendinoses (= Myotenones) in the:

T₁₂

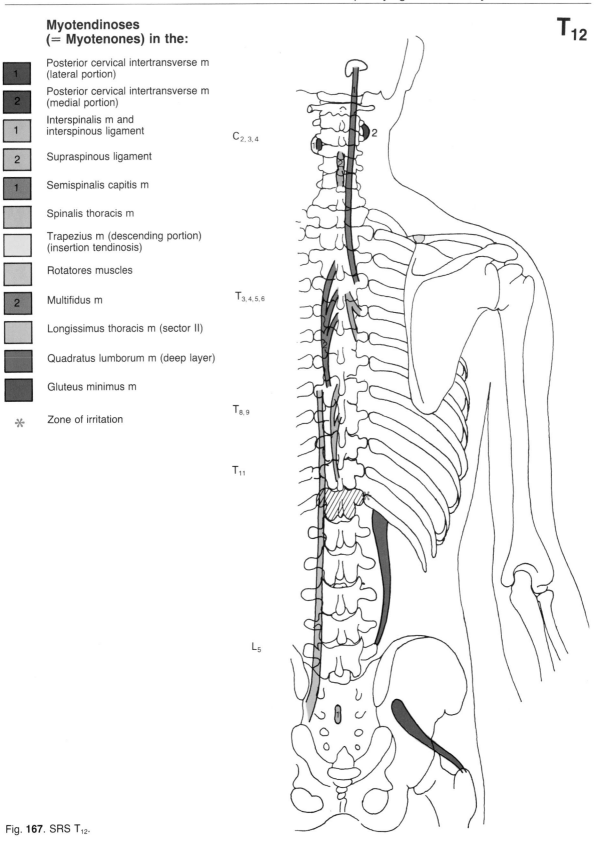

1	Posterior cervical intertransverse m (lateral portion)
2	Posterior cervical intertransverse m (medial portion)
1	Interspinalis m and interspinous ligament
2	Supraspinous ligament
1	Semispinalis capitis m
	Spinalis thoracis m
	Trapezius m (descending portion) (insertion tendinosis)
	Rotatores muscles
2	Multifidus m
	Longissimus thoracis m (sector II)
	Quadratus lumborum m (deep layer)
	Gluteus minimus m
*	Zone of irritation

$C_{2,3,4}$

$T_{3,4,5,6}$

$T_{8,9}$

T_{11}

L_5

Fig. **167**. SRS T_{12}.

**Myotendinoses
(= Myotenones) in the:**

L₁

1	Posterior cervical intertransverse m (lateral portion)
2	Posterior cervical intertransverse m (medial portion)
	Interspinales muscles
1	Semispinalis capitis m
	Trapezius m (horizontal portion)
	Rotatores muscles
2	Multifidus m
	Spinalis thoracis m
1	Longissimus thoracis m (sector II)
2	Longissimus thoracis m (sector III)
	Gluteus medius m (superficial layer)
	Gluteus maximus m (femoral portion)
✳	Zone of irritation

C₂,₃

C₃,₄

T₄,₅,₆

T₈

T₉

L₂,₃

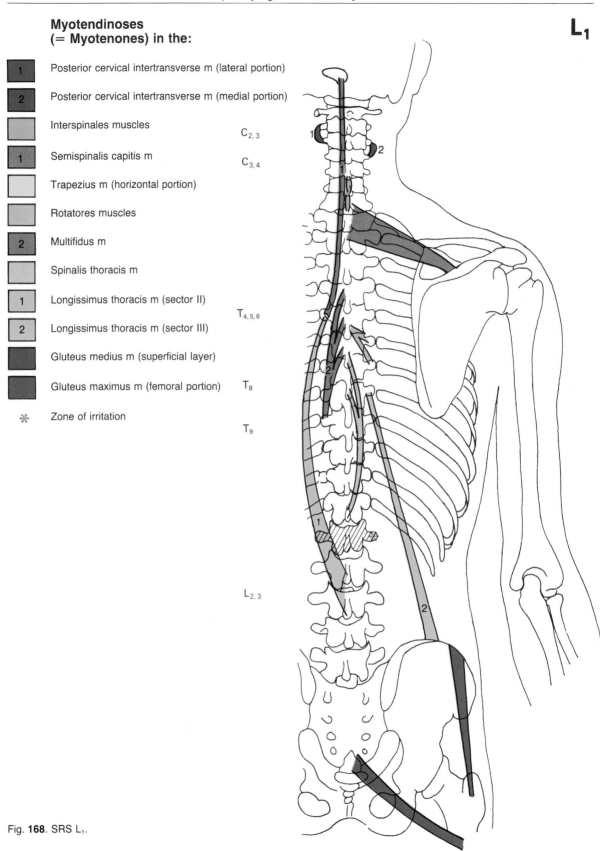

Fig. **168.** SRS L₁.

**Myotendinoses
(= Myotenones) in the:**

L₂

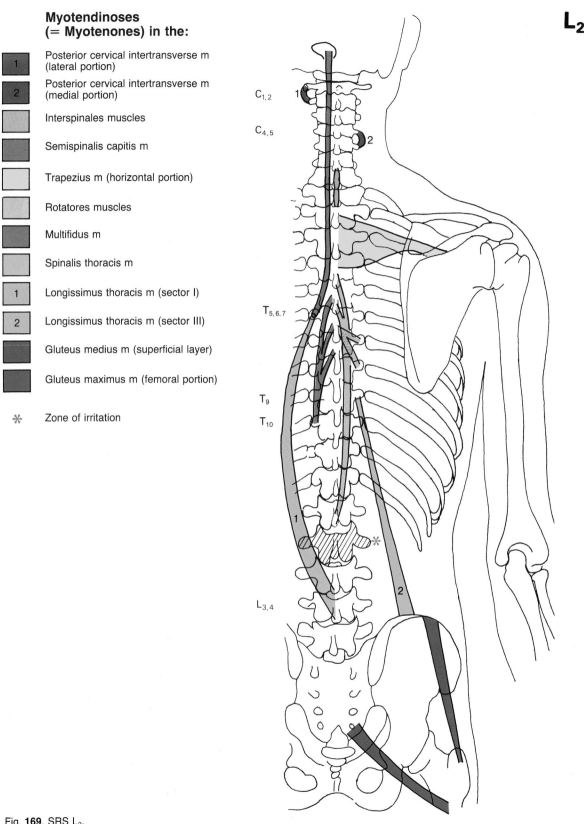

1	Posterior cervical intertransverse m (lateral portion)
2	Posterior cervical intertransverse m (medial portion)
	Interspinales muscles
	Semispinalis capitis m
	Trapezius m (horizontal portion)
	Rotatores muscles
	Multifidus m
	Spinalis thoracis m
1	Longissimus thoracis m (sector I)
2	Longissimus thoracis m (sector III)
	Gluteus medius m (superficial layer)
	Gluteus maximus m (femoral portion)
✳	Zone of irritation

Fig. **169**. SRS L₂.

**Myotendinoses
(= Myotenones) in the:**

L₃

1	Rectus capitis lateralis m
	Posterior cervical intertransverse m $C_{0,1}$
	Interspinales muscles
	Semispinalis capitis m $C_{4,5}$
2	
	Trapezius m (ascending portion)
	Rotatores muscles
3	Multifidus m
	Spinalis thoracis m
1	Longissimus thoracis m (sector I)
2	Longissimus thoracis m (sector III)
	Gluteus medius m (superficial layer) $T_{6,7,8}$
	Gluteus maximus m (femoral portion)
*	Zone of irritation

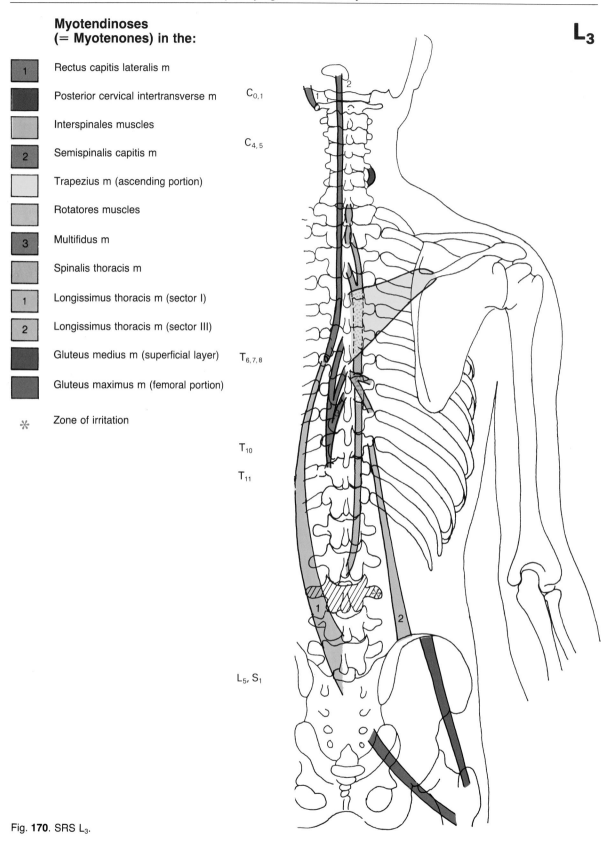

T_{10}

T_{11}

L_5, S_1

Fig. **170.** SRS L₃.

**Myotendinoses
(= Myotenones) in the:**

L₄

Posterior cervical intertransverse m

Interspinales muscles

Semispinalis capitis m

Trapezius m (ascending portion)

Rotatores muscles

Multifidus m

Spinalis thoracis m

Longissimus thoracis m (sector I)

Longissimus thoracis m (sector III)

Gluteus medius m (superficial layer)

Gluteus maximus m (femoral portion)

* Zone of irritation

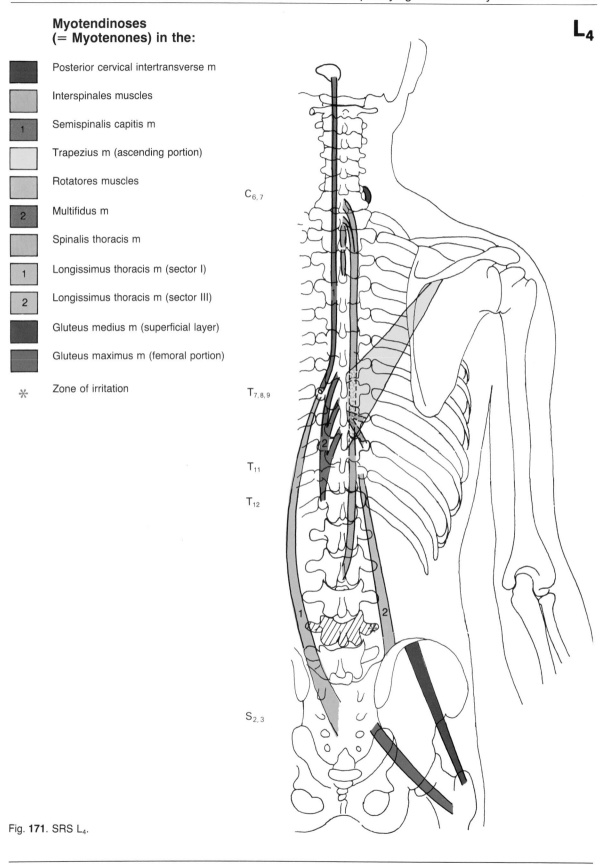

Fig. **171**. SRS L₄.

**Myotendinoses
(= Myotenones) in the:**

L$_5$

1   Rectus capitis posterior minor m

Posterior cervical intertransverse m   C$_{0,1}$

Interspinales mm

2   Iliocostalis cervicis m   C$_{3,4,5,6}$

Trapezius m (ascending portion)

C$_7$, T$_1$

Rotatores muscles

3   Multifidus m

1   Longissimus thoracis m (sector I)

2   Longissimus thoracis m (sector III)

Gluteus medius m (superficial layer)

Gluteus maximus m (femoral portion)

✳   Zone of irritation

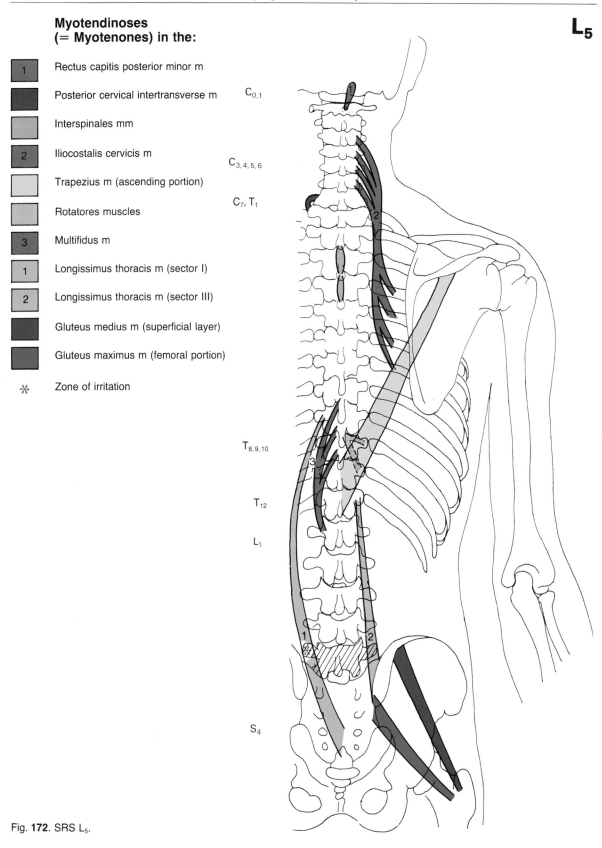

T$_{8,9,10}$

T$_{12}$

L$_1$

S$_4$

Fig. **172**. SRS L$_5$.

**Myotendinoses
(= Myotenones) in the:**

S₁

Rectus capitis posterior major m

1 Longissimus thoracis m (sector IV)

2 Longissimus lumborum m (lateral head)

Gluteus maximus m (tibial portion)

✳ Zone of irritation

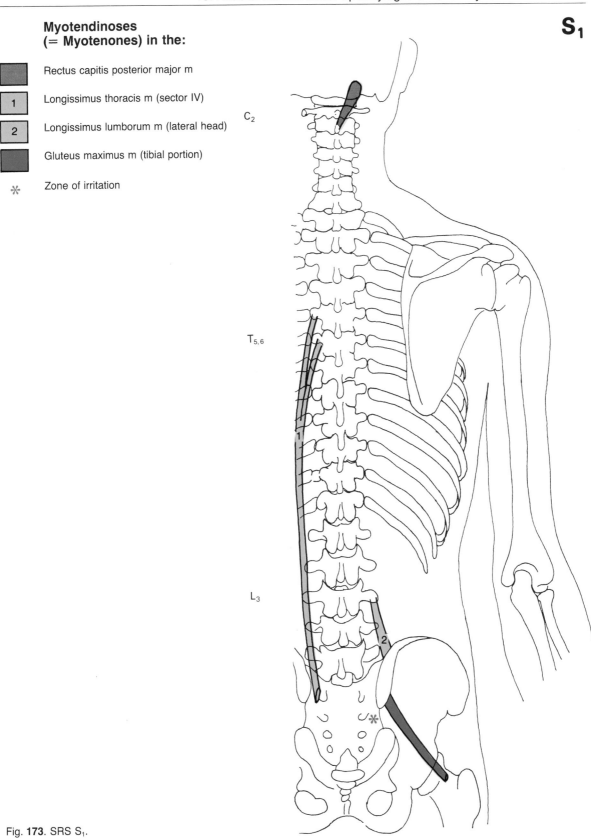

Fig. **173**. SRS S₁.

**Myotendinoses
(= Myotenones) in the:**

S_2

1   Longissimus thoracis m (sector IV)

2   Longissimus lumborum m (lateral head)

▪   Gluteus maximus m (tibial portion)

▪   Obliquus capitis inferior m

✳   Zone of irritation

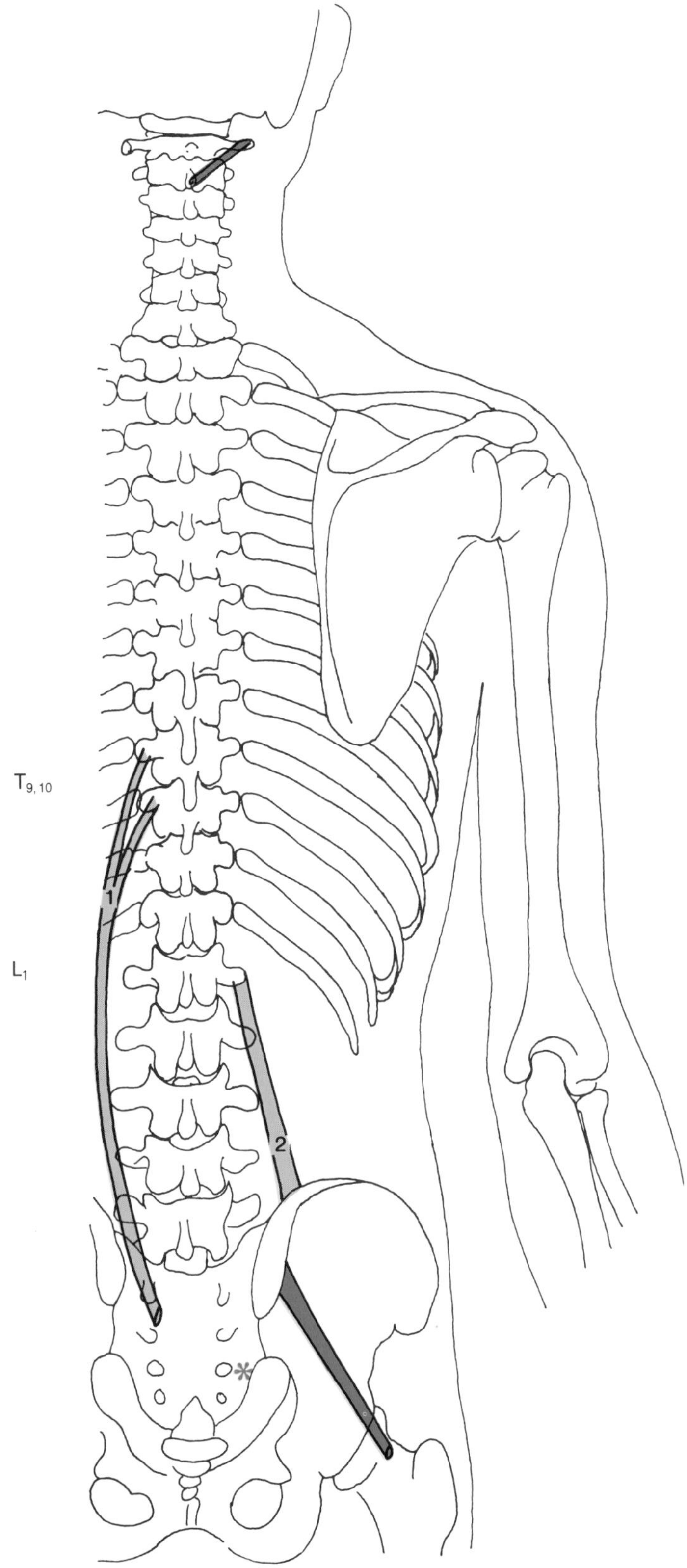

$T_{9,10}$

L_1

Fig. **174**. SRS S_2.

**Myotendinoses
(= Myotenones) in the:**

S₃

1   Longissimus thoracis m (sector IV)

2   Longissimus lumborum m (lateral head)

    Gluteus maximus m (tibial portion)

    Obliquus capitis superior m

*   Zone of irritation

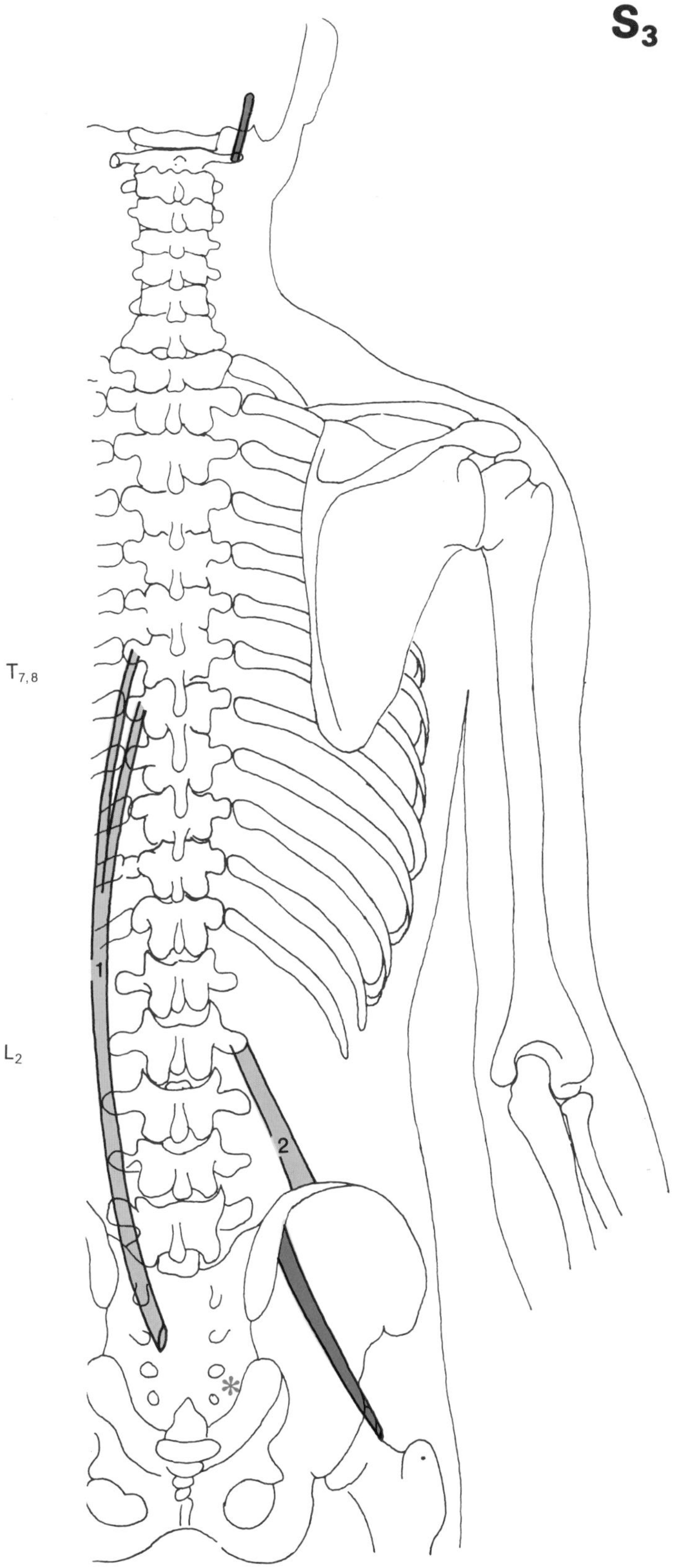

T₇,₈

L₂

Fig. **175**. SRS S₃.

Summary

Like every other scientific discipline, the field of medicine must remain open to new scientific accomplishments and developments. This applies to Manual Medicine as well.

This book attempts to summarize the present understanding of the spondylogenic reflex syndrome.

The spondylogenic correlation of individual myotenones described herein is the result of many years of experience. However, exceptions do exist, and new aspects can result in the change of spondylogenic correlations that have already been established for certain muscles pertaining to the axial skeleton. This would probably involve the quite small muscles or those muscles not easily accessible for palpation, such as the rotatores muscles, multifidus muscle, intertransverse and interspinales muscles. Further investigation is needed for a large number of peripheral muscles whose spondylogenic reflexogenic correlation has not been definitely determined.

While investigating the spondylogenic reflex syndrome, we came to the conclusion that one has to search for neurophysiological explanations that could help in the interpretation of these phenomena and thus scientifically substantiate the valuable clinical and empirical experiences.

References

Arnold, F.: Handbuch der Anatomie, vol 1, 1845.

Andriacchi, L. P., A. B. Schulz, T. B. Betrytsko, I. O. Galente: A model for studies of mechanical interactions between the thoracic spine and rib cage. J Biomech 7: 497, 1974.

Bernhard, W.: Kraniometrische Untersuchung zur funktionellen Morphologie des oberen Kopfgelenkes beim Menschen. Gegenbaurs Morphol Jahrb 122: 497, 1976.

Biemond, A., J. de Jong: On cervical nystagmus and related disorders. Brain 92: 437, 1969.

Bonica, J. J., D. Albe-Fessard: Advances in Pain Research and Therapy. Raven Press New York, 1980.

Borovansky, L.: Soustavna Anatomie Cloveka, 3. Aufl. SZN, Praha, 1967.

Brügger, A.: Über die Tendomyose. Dtsch Med. Wochenschr 83: 1048, 1958.

Brügger, A.: Vertebrale Syndrome. Acta rheumatol 18: 1, 1960.

Brügger, A.: Pseudoradikuläre Syndrome. Acta Rheumatol 19: 1, 1962.

Brügger, A.: Pseudoradikuläre Syndrome des Stammes. Huber, Bern, 1965.

Brügger, A.: Die Erkrankungen des Bewegungsapparates und seines Nervensystems. Fischer, Stuttgart, 1977.

Caviezel, H.: Beitrag zur Kenntnis der Rippenläsionen. Manuelle Med. 5: 110, 1974.

Caviezel, H.: Klinische Diagnostik der Funktionsstörung an den Kopfgelenken. Schweiz Rundsch Med Praxis 65 1037, 1976.

Depreux, R., H. Mestdagh: Anatomie fonctionelle de l'articulation sousoccipitale. Lille Méd 19: 122, 1974.

Dubs, R.: Beitrag zur Anatomie der lumbosakralen Region unter besonderer Berücksichtigung der Discushernie. Fortschr Neurol Psychiat 18: 69, 1950.

Dunbar, H., B. Ray: Chronic atlantoaxial dislocation with late neurologic manifestation. Surg Gynecol Obstet 113: 757, 1961.

Dvorak, J.: Rippenfrakturen. Dissertation. Zürich, 1976.

Dvorak, J.: Manuelle Medizin in USA in 1981. Manuelle Med 20: 1, 1982.

Dvorak, J., F. v. Orelli: Das Verhältnis der Komplikationen zu durchgeführten Manipulationen in der Schweiz. Schweiz Rundsch Med Praxis 71: 64, 1982.

Eisler, P.: Die Muskeln des Stammes. Fischer, Jena, 1912.

Fassbender, H. G.: Der rheumatische Schmerz. Med Welt 36: 1263, 1980.

Fassbender, H. G., K. Wegner: Morphologie und Pathogenese des Weichteilrheumatismus. Rheumaforschung 32: 355, 1973.

Feinstein, B., J. N. K. Langton, R. M. Jameson, F. Schitter: Experiments on pain referred from deep somatic tissues. J Bone Joint Surg 36A: 981, 1954.

Fielding, J. W.: Cineroentgenography of the normal cervical spine. J. Bone Joint Surg 39A: 1280, 1957.

Fielding, J. W.: Spine fusion for atlanto axial instability. J Bone Joint Surg 58A: 400, 1976.

Fielding, J. W., G. V. B. Cochron, J. F. Lansing III, M. Hohl: Tears of the transverse ligament of the atlas. J Bone Joint Surg 56A: 8, 1974.

Fielding, J. W., R. J. Hawkins, R. N. Hensinger, W. R. Francis: Deformities. Orthop Clin North Am 9: 955, 1978.

Freeman, M. A. R., B. D. Wyke: The innervation of the knee joint. An anatomical and histological study in the cat. J Anat 101: 505, 1967.

Frigerio, N.: Movement of the sacroiliac joints. Clin Orthop 100: 370, 1974.

Gerstenbrand, F., H. Tilscher, M. Berger: Radikuläre und pseudoradikuläre Symptome der mittleren und unteren Halswirbelsäule. Münch Med. Wochenschr 121: 1173, 1979.

Gibson, R. W.: The evolution of chiropractic. In Haldeman, S.: Modern Developments in the Principles and Practice of Chiropractic. Appleton-Century-Crofts, New York, 1980.

Glen, W. V., M. L. Rhodes, E. M. Altschuler, L. L. Wiltse, C. Kostanek, Y. M. Kuo: Multi planar display computerized body tomography applications in the lumbar spine. Spine 4: 108, 1979.

Goldstein, M.: The research status of spinal manipulative therapy. 1975 National Institute of Neurological and Communicating Disorders and Stroke, Monograph, No. 15, US. Department of Health, Education, and Welfare, Publication No. (National Institutes of Health) 76–998, 1976.

Granit, R., O. Pompeiano: Reflex control of posture and movement. Progr Brain Res 50: 1, 1979.

Gutzeit, K.: Der vertebrale Faktor im Krankheitsgeschehen Manuelle Med 19: 66, 1981.

Hikosaka, O., M. Maeda: Cervical effect on abducens motoneurones and their interaction with the vestibulo-ocular reflex. Exp Brain Res 18: 512, 1973.

Hockaday, J. M., C. W. M. Whitty: Patterns of referred pain in normal subject. Brain 90: 481, 1967.

Hohermuth, H. J.: Spondylogene Kniebeschwerden. Vortrag anläßlich der 4. Deutsch-Schweizerischen Fortbildungstagung für Angiologie und Rheumatologie. Rheinfelden, Mai 1981

Hohl, M., H. Baker: The atlanto-axial joint. J. Bone Joint Surg 46A: 1739, 1964.

Hoover, R. V.: Functional technic. Yearbook, Academy of Applied Osteopathy. Carmel, Cal., 1958 p 47.

Igarashi, M., H. Miyata, B. R. Alford, W. K. Wright: Nystagmus after experimental cervical laesion. Laryngoscope 82: 1609, 1972.

Ingelmark, B. E.: Ueber den craniocervicalen Uebergang beim Menschen. Acta Anat. [Suppl] 6: 1, 1949.

Jayson, M. I. V.: The Lumbar Spine and Back Pain, 2nd ed. Pitman, London, 1980.

Jirout, J.: Changes in the atlas-axis relations on lateral flexion of the head and neck. Neuroradiology 6: 215, 1973.

Jones, L. M.: Spontaneous release by positioning. Doctor of Osteopathy 4: 109, 1964.

Jones, L. M.: Strain and Counterstrain. The American Academy of Osteopathy, Colorado Springs, 1981.

De Jong, P. T. V. M., J. M. B. Vianney, B. Cochen, L. B. W. Jongkees: Ataxia and nystagmus induced by injection of local anaesthetics in the neck. Ann Neurol 1: 240, 1977.

Keller, H. M., W. E. Meier, D. A. Kumpe: Noninvasive angiography for the diagnosis of vertebral artery disease using Dopplerultrasound. Stroke 7: 364, 1976.

Kellgren, J. H.: Observation of referred pain arising from muscles. Clin Sci 3: 175, 1938.

Kellgren, J. H.: On the distribution of pain arising from deep somatic structures with charts of segmental pain areas. Clin Sci 4: 35, 1939.

Kennedy, J. C., R. J. Hawkins, R. B. Willis, K. D. Danylchuck: Tension studies of human knee ligaments. J Bone Joint Surg 58A: 350, 1976.

Knese, K.: Kopfgelenk, Kopfhaltung und Kopfbewegung des Menschen. Z Anat Entwickl-Gesch 114: 67, 1947/50.

Korr, I. M.: Proprioceptors and somatic dysfunction. J Am Osteopath Assoc 74: 638, 1975.

v. Lanz, T., W. Wachsmuth: Praktische Anatomie, Vol. I. part 1, Springer, Berlin, 1979.

Lewis, T., J. H. Kellgren: Observations relating to referred pain viscero-motor reflexes and other associated phenomena. Clin Sci 4: 47, 1939.

Lewit, K.: Blockierung von Atlas-Axis und Atlas-Occiput im Rö-Bild und Klinik. Z Orthop 108: 43, 1970.

Lewit, K.: Manuelle Medizin im Rahmen der medizinischen Rehabilitation. Urban & Schwarzenberg, München, 1977.

Lewit, K.: Muskelfazilitations- und Inhibitionstechniken in der Manuellen Medizin. Manuelle Med 19: 12, 1981.

Ludwig, K.: Über das Lig. alare dentis. Z Anat Entwickl-Gesch 116: 442, 1952.

Lumsden, R. M., J. M. Morris: An in vivo study of axial rotation and immobilization at the lumbosacral joint. J Bone Joint Surg 50A: 1591, 1968.

Lysell, E.: Motion in the cervical spine. Acta Orthop Scand [Suppl] 123: 1, 1969.

Macalister, A.: Notes on the development and variations of the atlas. J Anat Physiol 27: 518, 1893.

Maigne, R.: Wirbelsäulenbedingte Schmerzen. Hippokrates, Stuttgart, 1970.

Melzack, R.: Phantom body pain in paraplegics: Evidence for central "pattern generating mechanism" for pain. Pain 4: 195, 1978.

Melzack, R.: Myofascial trigger points: relation to acupuncture and mechanisms of pain. Arch Phys Med 62: 114, 1981.

Memorandum der Deutschen Gesellschaft für Manuelle Medizin: Zur Verhütung der Zwischenfälle bei gezielter Handgriff-Therapie an der HWS. Manuelle Med 17: 53, 1979

Mitchell, F. L., P. S. Moran, N. A. Pruzzo: An Evaluation and Treatment Manual of Osteopathic Muscle Energy Procedures. Mitchell, Moran, Pruzzo, Valley Park, Mo., 1979.

Mixter, W. J., J. S. Barr: Rupture of intervertebral disc with involvement of spinal canal. N Engl J Med 211: 210, 1934.

Molina, F., J. E. Ramcharan, B. D. Wyke: Structure and function of articular receptor system in the cervical spine. J Bone Joint Surg. 58B: 255, 1976.

Moll, J. M., V. Wright: Normal range of spinal mobility. Ann Rheum. Dis 30: 387, 1971.

Mumenthaler, M.: Der Schulter-Arm-Schmerz. Huber, Bern, 1981.

Mumenthaler, M., H. Schliack: Läsion der peripheren Nerven, 3. ed. Thieme, Stuttgart, 1977.

Northup, G. W.: Osteopathic Medicine: An American Reformation. American Osteopathic Association, Chicago, 1966.

Panjabi, M. M., J. Hausfeld, A. White: Experimental determination of thoracic spine stability. Presented at the 24th annual meeting of Orthopaedic Research Society, Dallas, 1978.

Penning, L.: Functional pathology of the cervical spine. Excerpta Medica Foundation, Amsterdam, 1968.

Perl, E.: Pain, spinal and peripheral nerve factors. 1975 National Institute of Neurological and Communicative Disorders and Stroke. Monograph 173–185, 1975.

Reynolds, M. D.: Myofascial trigger point syndromes in the practice of rheumatology. Arch Phys. Med 62: 111, 1981

Richmond, F. J., V. C. Abrahams: What are the proprioceptors of the neck? Prog Brain Res 50: 245, 1979.

Rubin, D.: Myofascial trigger point syndromes: An approach to management. Arch Phys Med 62: 107, 1981.

Sato, A.: The somato-sympathetic reflexes: Their physiological and clinical significance. 1975 National Institute of Neurological and Communicative Disorders and Stroke. Monograph No. 15, 163–172.

Schmid, H.: Das Iliosacralgelenk in einer Untersuchung mit Röntgenstereophotogrammetrie und einer klinischen Studie. Akt Rheumatol 5: 163, 1980.

Schmorl, G., H. Junghanns: Die gesunde und die kranke Wirbelsäule in Röntgenbild und Klinik, 5. ed. Thieme, Stuttgart, 1968.

Schulz, A. B., D. Benson, O. Hirsch: Force deformation properties of human ribs. J Biomech 7: 303, 1974.

Schulz, A. B., D. Benson, O. Hirsch: Force deformation properties of human costosternal and costovertebral articulations. J Biomech 7: 311, 1974.

Schwarz, E.: Manuelle Medizin und innere Medizin. Schweiz Rundsch Med (Praxis) 63: 837, 1974.

Sell, K.: Spezielle manuelle Segment-Technik als Mittel zur Abklärung spondylogener Zusammenhangsfragen. Manuelle Med 7: 99, 1969.

Selvik, G.: A Roentgen stereophotogrammetric method for the study of the kinematics of the sceletal system. AV-Centralen, Lund, 1974.

Simons, D. G.: Electrogenic nature of palpable bands and local twitch response associated with myofascial trigger points. In Bonica, J. J., D. Albe-Fessard: Advances in Pain Research and Therapy, vol. I. Raven Press, New York, 1976.

Simons, D. G.: Muscle pain syndromes. Am Phys Med 54: 289, 1975; 55: 15, 1976.

Sinclair, D. C., W. H. Feindel, G. Weddell, M. A. Falconer: The intervertebral ligaments as a source of segmental pain. J Bone Joint Surg 30B: 515, 1948.

Steel, H.: Anatomical and mechanical consideration of the atlanto-axial articulation. J Bone Joint Surg 50A: 1481, 1968.

Stoff, E.: Zur Morphometrie der Gelenkflächen des oberen Kopfgelenkes. Verh Anat Ges (Jena) 70: 575, 1976.

Sutter, M.: Versuch einer Wesensbestimmung pseudoradiku-
lärer Syndrome. Schweiz Rundsch Med Praxis 63: 842, 1974.

Sutter, M.: Wesen, Klinik und Bedeutung spondylogener
Reflexsyndrome. Schweiz Rundsch Med Praxis 64: 42, 1975.

Sutter, M.: Rückern-, Kreuz- und Beinschmerzen bei funk-
tionell instabilen Becken. Ther Umsch 34: 452, 1977.

Sutter, M., R. Fröhlich: Spondylogene Zusammenhänge im
Bereiche der oberen Thorax-Apparatur. Report of the Annual Meeting of the Swiss Society for Manual Medicine,
1981.

Travell, J.: Myofascial trigger points: Clinical view. In Bonica,
J. J., D. G. Albe-Fessard: Advances in Pain Research and
Therapy, vol. I. Raven Press, New York, 1976 p. 199.

Travell, J.: Identification of myofascial trigger point syndromes: a case of atypical facial neuralgia. Arch Phys Med
62: 100, 1981.

Travell, J., S. H. Rinzler: The myofascial genesis of pain.
Postgrad Med 2: 425, 1952.

Vrettos, X. C., B. Wyke: Articular reflexogenic systems in the
costovertebral joints. J Bone Joint Surg 56B: 382, 1979.

Waller, U.: Pathogenese des spondylogenen Reflexsyndroms.
Schweiz Rundsch Med Praxis 64: 42, 1975.

Walther, D. S.: Applied Kinesiology. SDC System, Pueblo
Col, 1981.

Wardwell, W. I.: The present and future role of the chiroprac-
tor. In Haldeman, S.: Modern Developments in the Princi-
pals and Practice of Chiropractic. Appleton Century-Crofts,
New York, 1980.

Werne, S.: Studies in spontaneous atlas dislocation. Acta
Orthop Scand [Suppl] 23: 1, 1957.

White, A., M. M. Panjabi: The basic kinematics of the human
spine. Spine 3: 13, 1978a.

White, A., M. M. Panjabi: Clinical Biomechanics of the Spine.
Lippincott, Philadelphia, 1978b.

Wolf-Heidegger, G.: Atlas der systematischen Anatomie des
Menschen. Karger, Basel, 1961.

Wyke, B. D.: The neurological basis of thoracic spinal pain.
Rheum Phys. Med 10: 356, 1967.

Wyke, B. D.: Morphological and functional features of the
innervation of the costovertebral joints. Folia Morphol 23:
296, 1975.

Wyke, B. D.: Clinical significance of articular receptor system
in the limbs and spine. Proc. of the 5th Int. Congress of
Manual Medicine, Copenhagen, 1977.

Wyke, B. D.: Neurological mechanisms in the experience of
pain. Acupuncture and Electro-Ther Res 4: 27, 1979a.

Wyke, B. D.: Neurology of the cervical spinal joints.
Physiotherapy 65: 72, 1979b.

Wyke, B. D.: Perspectives in physiotherapy. Physiotherapy
32: 261, 1980.

Wyke, B. D., P. Polacek: Structural and functional characteristics of the joint receptor apparatus. Acta Chir Orthop
Traum. Čech. 40: 489, 1973.

Wyke, B. D., P. Polacek: Articular neurology – the present
position. J Bone Joint Surg 57B: 401, 1975.

Index